MELATONIN
in health and
disease

Ismail Gögenur

Jacob Rosenberg

Remember, life is a game you cannot win, but play it with gusto!!

CONTENTS

PREFACE

Twenty years ago, at the department of surgery, we discussed the issue of sleep problems in patients after surgery. We had noticed that a great proportion of our patients did not sleep well and in addition had a disturbed daily rhythm with a lot of sleeping during the daytime and wake periods during the night. We also found out that the typical time of unexpected death would be in the early morning hours compared with other times during the day. We therefore asked ourselves if there were troubles with the internal clock and hence we got interested in the hormone melatonin.

We found out in several studies, that patients had a kind of "jet-lag" after surgery and treatment with melatonin might be helping stabilizing their daily rhythms. When we started doing this research there were new reports regarding the potent other effects of melatonin such as its antioxidant effect. A lot of our patients have a high degree of oxidative stress after surgery and we hypothesized that this potent endogenous antioxidant would help these patients in reducing their risk of getting cardiac complications in the postoperative period. We could show this in the next studies and it was as if there were more and more fields of research where melatonin was a highly relevant substance and drug to consider.

For over 20 years we have made several research projects within this field and in this book we are summing up the various important implications of treating patients with melatonin. In addition, and at least as important, we also go through the many interesting studies that have shown an effect of melatonin as a supplement to prevent certain diseases. As it can be seen in this book there are some very interesting perspectives of melatonin treatment in frequent diseases such as hypertension, heart disease, diabetes and cancer. It has been a tremendous interesting journey to write this book and we hope that the readers will have a good understanding of what melatonin is all about - in health and disease!

PHYSIOLOGY/INTRODUCTION

What is melatonin

Melatonin is a hormone, which has drawn the interest of an increasing number of scientists and healthcare professionals around the world in the recent 30 to 40 years. Parallel to this development, this versatile hormone has also the attention of people around the world that use this hormone in their daily life as a supplement to stay healthy, as a sleeping aid or as a pill that they are taking when travelling long distance by airplane. Approximately 8 million people in the United States are taking melatonin on a regular basis for various reasons. As it will be presented in the following chapters, this interesting hormone has some intriguing effects with a potential huge importance for preventing serious diseases in the brain, heart, kidneys, sleep disturbances, circadian disturbances, and actually also in the prevention and treatment of cancer. An important aspect about melatonin is that it can be taken in very high doses without producing any kind of side effects. In the recent couple of years it has also been shown, that melatonin has an extremely interesting and powerful effect for prevention of situations where the human body is under acute stress. In addition, melatonin has also shown to play a central role in the development of some of the most important health issues posing a threat to millions of patients worldwide. A clear example of this is the newly discovered relationship between melatonin and the development of diabetes.

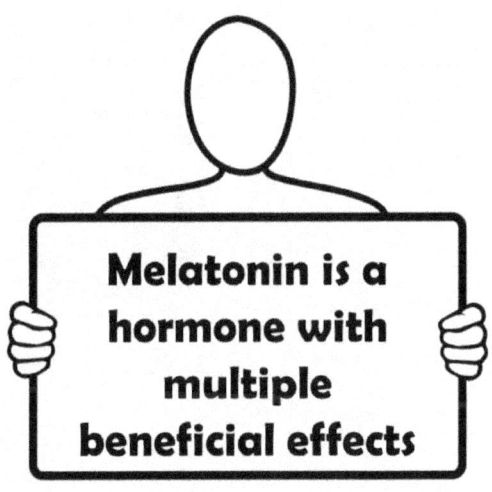

How is it possible to have a hormone that plays such a central role in so many different basic body functions and in so many disease processes? One way to understand this is to have a look on what kinds of organ systems and tissues utilize or produce melatonin in their normal function. The main place where melatonin is produced in the human body is in the center of the brain. This production site is called the pineal gland.

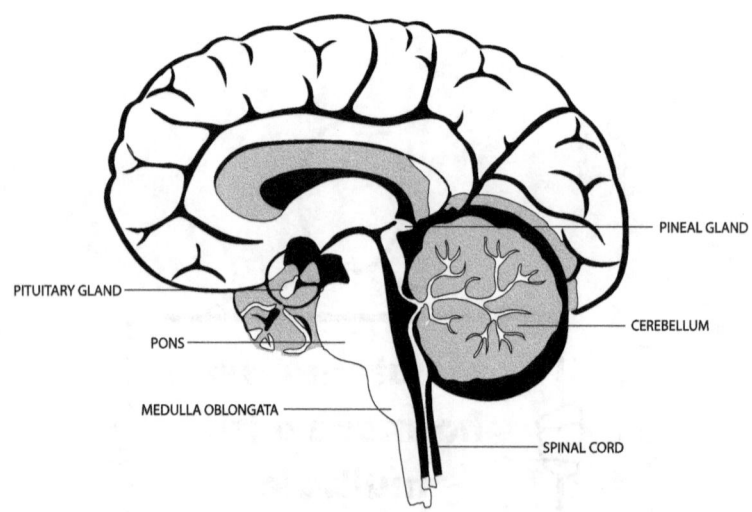

The prominent Greek physician, surgeon and philosopher in the Roman Empire Claudius Gallenius known as Galen of Pergamon made the first description of the pineal gland and its location in the human brain. This Greek physician had a great interest in the anatomy of the human brain, and he gave the name to this pineal gland for its pine and cone shape. This was in the years approximately 200 AD. Much later the famous French philosopher and mathematician René Descartes described that the pineal gland was the "seat of the sole". Descartes saw the pineal gland as a place where the psychology and the physiology were connected. It was only in 1948 that the American professor Aaron B Lerner discovered that the main hormone produced by the pineal gland was in fact melatonin. The name melatonin was given based on the interesting observations from professor Lerner that when adding pineal extract to frog skin it induced a color change with lightening of the frog's skin.

Basic functions of melatonin

Melatonin is secreted by the pineal gland with a circadian rhythm. A circadian rhythm means that the rhythm varies according to the solar day (24 hours approximately). The secretion of melatonin is maximal during the nighttime with a peak in the production between 2 am and 4 am. If a person lives in a place where there are longer nights, this is also reflected as a longer duration of a high concentration of melatonin in the blood. Thus, melatonin is a signal of darkness that is a code for time of day and length of day information to the brain and other organs. This very tight regulation of melatonin from the pineal gland is controlled by another center in the brain called the suprachiasmatic nucleus. This small collection of nerves receives information from the eyes with specific information about the light levels in the environment. In other words, if there is light stimulation to the eyes due to sun exposure or staying inside in a place where there is artificial light, the brain receives information that it should not secrete melatonin from the pineal gland. As soon as the light levels are reduced in the evening hours, than the increase of melatonin begins.

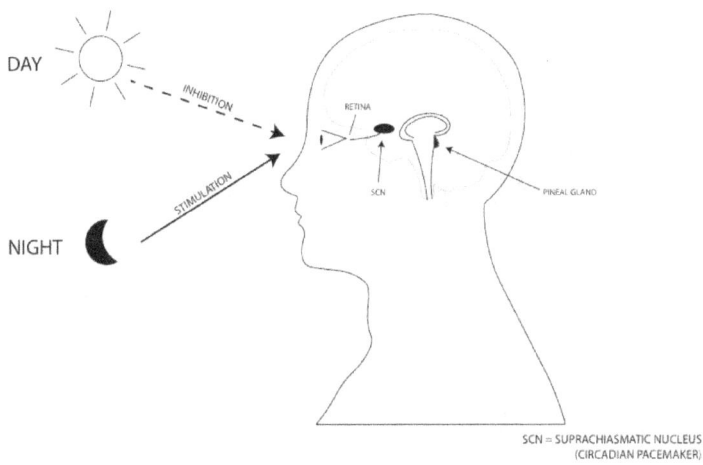

SCN = SUPRACHIASMATIC NUCLEUS
(CIRCADIAN PACEMAKER)

The circadian regulation of bodily rhythms is highly dependent on light in the surroundings.

The opposite correlation also exists because taking melatonin can actually shift circadian rhythms in humans. For example in blind persons a dose of melatonin ranging from 0.5 to 5 mg can regulate the circadian rhythm even when there is no possibility for seeing from the light in the environment due to blindness.

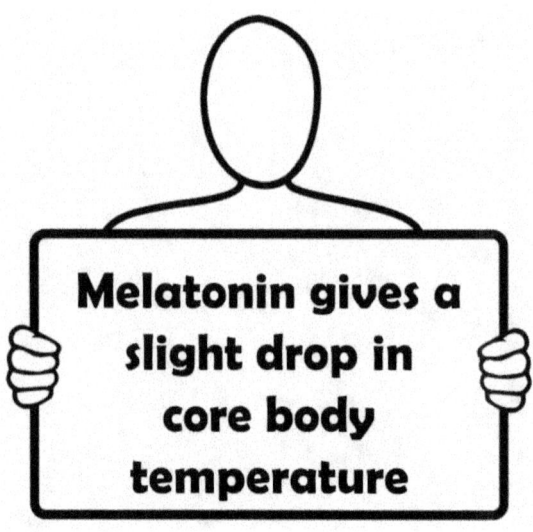

Having a hormone that is so tightly regulated to nighttime must also have an effect on sleep. This is certainly the case, because there is a very tight regulation between the need to sleep and the melatonin increase in blood in the evening hours. When melatonin increases in the evening hours the core body temperature drops. This results in a signal telling the brain that now it is time to sleep. This is why melatonin is also known to be the hormone that "opens the sleep gate". This actually also means that, if melatonin is taken in daytime where the concentration of melatonin in the blood is very low, it can have sleep inducing effects by lowering body temperature and inducing fatigue.

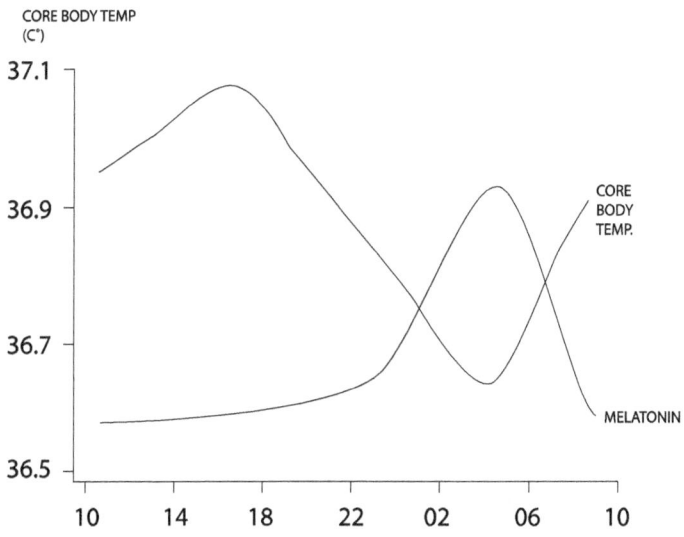

Melatonin rises in the evening hours at the same time as the core body temperature drops.

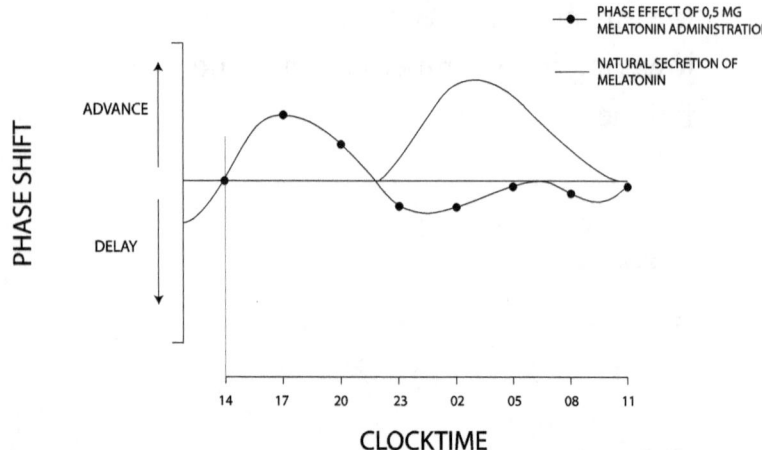

If melatonin is administered in the afternoon it results in phase advance meaning that the circadian rhythms are peaking earlier than planned and the opposite when melatonin is administered in the night-time and early morning.

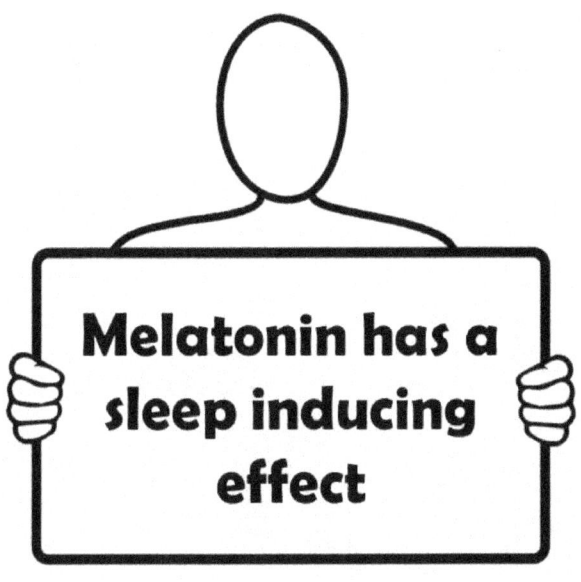

The concentration of melatonin in blood is also different in the elderly, where it is shown, that as a person gets older, there is a decrease in the concentration of melatonin in the blood during the night, and this actually may be an explaining factor for sleep problems in the elderly. The concentration of melatonin is much higher in early life.

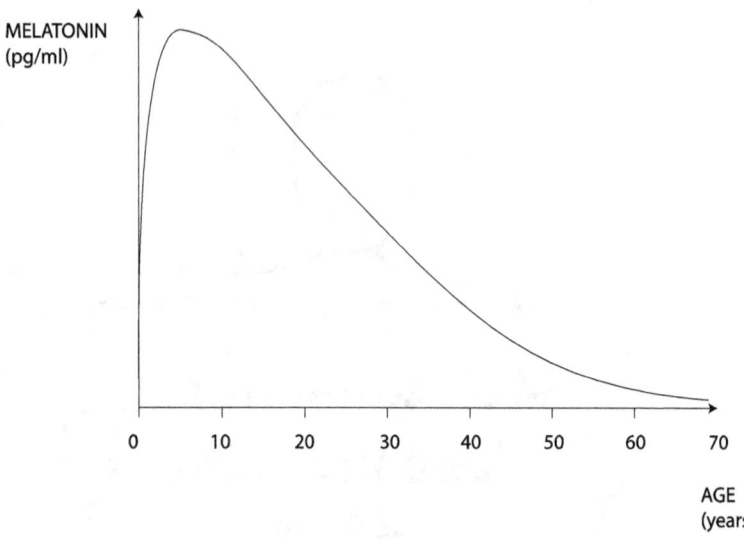

High concentrations of melatonin are seen in childhood, decreasing in adulthood and lowest levels are seen in the elderly.

Within the last 20 to 30 years there have been numerous studies showing that melatonin is one of the most effective antioxidants in the human body. An antioxidant is a substance that blocks the damaging effects of the so-called free radicals. These free radicals are molecules characterized by a high potential of damaging other molecules or cell structures. It is believed that the constant generation of free radicals that are produced in human cells and which are not blocked or detoxified can result in various conditions such as chronic brain diseases, heart diseases and cancer. The natural question to ask would then be: Is there an increased risk of cancer if there is a continued low production of

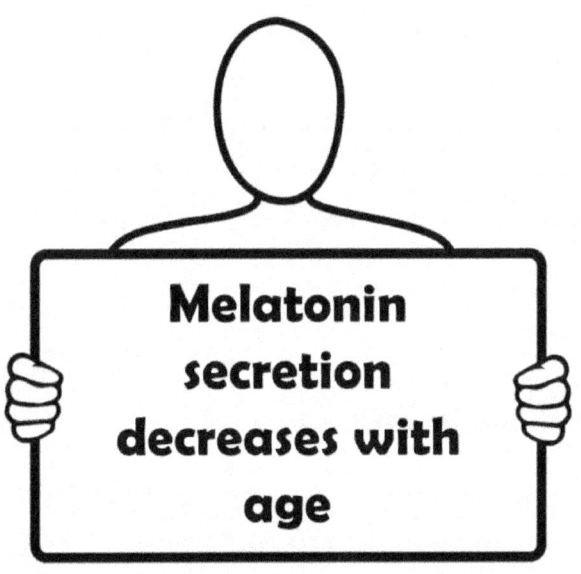

Melatonin secretion decreases with age

melatonin during the night? This has been investigated in shift workers. Due to the constant exposure to artificial light during the night, shift workers do not have a high concentration of melatonin during the night. It has been shown, that if the melatonin concentration is low during the night and there are more than four to five of these "no melatonin nights" due to shift work, this will result in an increased risk of cancer. Thus, nurses that work more than four to five nights during one month and have a continuous work schedule like this has an increased risk of breast cancer.

The above mentioned fascinating effects of melatonin in health and disease will be described in more details in the following chapters.

Melatonin in nature

The first time researchers found melatonin in plants was in 1993. The researchers found concentrations of melatonin in tomato fruits and two years later, there were additional reports showing, that melatonin was present in other eatable plants as well. Within the last 15 to 20 years, it has been shown, that there are melatonin in different eatables such as kiwi fruit, pineapple, asparagus, spinach, rice seed, banana, apple, grape, wine and red wine and in sun flower seeds. The concentration of melatonin is highly variable in these eatables.

Eatable plants / fruits	Concentration (pg/g)
Asparagus	9.5
Cucumber fruit seed	24.6
Rice seed	1006
Sweet corn	1366
Kiwi	24.4
Banana	0.46
Apple	47.6
Carrot	55.3
Red wine	200 (pg/mL)

10 eatable plants/fruits with different melatonin concentrations.

The physiological role of melatonin in the function of plants is believed to be of mainly regulatory character where the melatonin inside the plant regulates the growth of different parts of the plant. In addition, it is believed, that due to melatonin's antioxidant effect, it can reduce degradation of leaves and thus result in longevity of the plants. What is very intriguing is, that melatonin in plants may also have a light and dark cycle. It has been shown, that the concentration of melatonin varies according to the light environment. Thus, melatonin may be an important signal for circadian changes in plant functions.

Of major interest in the future regarding the functions of melatonin, is its possibility to prevent the damaging effects of chemical agents. It has been shown that, if there is copper in the soil, or herbicides, or UV radiation, the presence of melatonin can prevent the damaging effect of these. It is therefore proposed, that melatonin may have a role in the future to protect plants in an environment where there is industrial waste or soil containing waste products from agricultural use.

Melatonin metabolites and receptors

Melatonin is a substance that is both soluble in water and in lipids. This means that it can be distributed into almost all tissues in the human body. There is a great variation in the secretion of melatonin from subject to subject, thus some may have only 10 micrograms of melatonin in the blood at their maximum during the night and others may have 80 micrograms at their maximum level during the night. For the individual subject, there is much less variation and the melatonin rhythm is very robust. After melatonin has been secreted into the blood, the main site clearing the melatonin is the liver. The liver clears more than 90% of circulating melatonin and the major metabolites are excreted in the urine.

When hormones are secreted into the blood they induce changes in cells by primarily molecules called receptors in the surface of the cells. When a hormone is placed on a receptor it induces a change in the cellular function. This is also the case for melatonin as it has been shown, that there are different melatonin receptors in different tissues around the body. Besides the effect that melatonin induces through receptors, it is also known that melatonin goes through the cell membranes and changes the function of proteins and receptors inside the cells. This factor has been drawing a lot of attention because it has been shown that melatonin is secreted in many different tissues and cells such as the glands that produce tears, red blood cells, immune cells and in the intestines. Especially the presence of melatonin in the intestines is believed to have an important function in the immune response. Melatonin is believed to block the deleterious effects of bacteria that pass through the bowel wall and into the blood stream. It is then the antioxidant effects that help killing the bacteria that enters the blood stream.

When antioxidants results in a protective effect, they can eliminate one free radical and then the molecule that it is converted to in this process, does not have any further protective effects. This is not the case for melatonin. When melatonin is converted to different compounds, these compounds have further antioxidant effects as well. Actually, some of the metabolites are more active than melatonin itself. This is the case of melatonin in the skin.

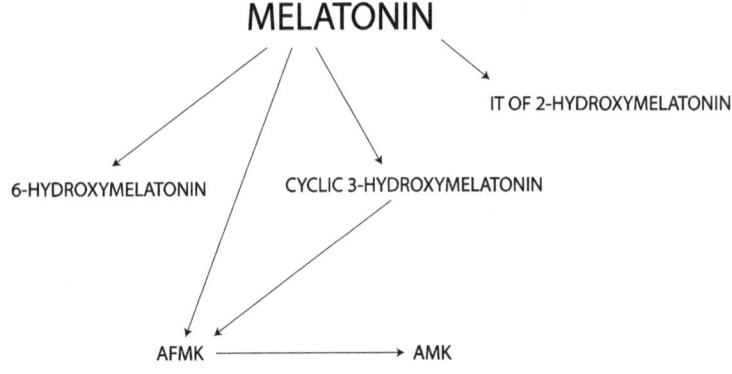

Different metabolites in the metabolism of melatonin. Most metabolites have high antioxidant properties.

MELATONIN FOR TREATMENT OF CIRCADIAN RHYTHM AND SLEEP DISORDERS

Many patients suffer from a condition belonging to a group of diseases called circadian rhythm sleep disorders. These disorders all involve a problem in the timing of when a person sleeps and is awake. It is a result of a non-functioning internal "body clock" or a mismatch between the internal body clock and the environment. When a person is suffering from this kind of mismatch between the internal clock and the environment, he or she will have complaints of poor sleep at certain times and too much sleepiness at other times of the day. This usually results in difficulties in a person's work, school, or in social relations.

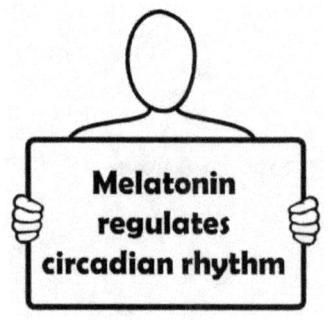

Delayed sleep phase disorder

This is a condition, which usually is seen in adults and adolescents. It is believed, that there is about 0.2% to 10% of a population, which suffers from this disorder. Milder cases are luckily more prevalent. There is a genetic component of the disease and in certain patients it is seen more often than in others. For example, if a patient has cirrhosis, which is a situation where there is reduced liver function, these patients are having higher risk of developing delayed sleep phase disorder. The usual pattern of adults with this condition is the so called "night owl", staying up late, usually until 2-3 am and waking up late at noon or even later, if they are allowed to sleep. If these youngsters are forced to wake up earlier, this may result in poor school performance due to sleepiness in the daytime or even work accidents. Due to this pattern of sleep, these persons are often regarded as slow, unmotivated or lazy.

Melatonin is very effective in treating this disorder, and it is recommended that it is taken at certain times in the afternoon in order to advance the sleepiness and the circadian rhythm. Taking 0.5 to 5 mg of melatonin results in an effective treatment of the symptoms and stabilization of the circadian rhythm. If the patients stop taking melatonin almost all patients relapse within few days to few months, so it is necessary with chronic treatment with melatonin. Besides melatonin it is also effective to give bright light therapy in the daytime. Melatonin treatment is also effective in preventing depression in youngsters suffering from delayed sleep phase syndrome.

Advanced sleep phase disorder

Advanced sleep disorder is less common than delayed sleep phase disorder with prevalence in the population of approximately 1%. It usually starts to affect patients in the elderly and age may be a risk factor for this condition.

Advanced sleep phase disorder is a

situation, when a person regularly goes to sleep, but wakes much earlier than most people. Thus, it is obvious to name these patients as "morning types" who typically will be waking up between 2 and 5 am, but also go to sleep early in the evening between 6 pm until 9 pm. It is characteristic that, if you allow a person with advanced sleep phase disorder to go to sleep at preferred time and wake up at preferred time, they will have a regular and stable sleep pattern. In this condition it has been shown, that treatment with melatonin administered in the early morning hours will advance the circadian phase and melatonin may also be used for difficulties maintaining sleep.

Irregular sleep-wake rhythm disorder

Irregular sleep-wake rhythm disorder is primarily seen in the elderly and especially in patients with Alzheimer's disease. This condition has also been shown to be prevalent in patients after a major trauma or in children with developmental disorders.

The characteristics of irregular sleep-wake rhythm disorder, is that these patients suffer from several short intervals of 1 to 4 hours of sleep during 24 hours. The longest period is seen in the mid-night period. In total, the patients are actually sleeping a normal duration of sleep. Thus, these patients greatest problem is a severely fragmental sleep and many daytime naps. This results in sleepiness during the daytime and difficulties maintaining sleep. It has been shown, that if melatonin is given at bedtime and is combined with light during the day, that these patients will have relief of symptoms. Doses between 2-20 mg have shown effects in children with this condition.

None-24-hours sleep-wake disorder

None-24-hours sleep-wake disorder is a condition when the circadian rhythm is not entrained to the environment and it is also called "free running rhythm disorder". This condition is prevalent mostly in blind people, and almost 50% of these have this condition. It can also be seen in sighted people but this is much less common. There is a male predominance of approximately 3 males to 1 female having this condition. Due to the free running characteristic, the symptoms depend on when the person is required to sleep. Because the internal rhythm is free running and typically has a daily drift to later and later times, the patient will have symptoms of poor sleep and daytime sleepiness for several weeks. Thus, there will also be days to weeks where there are no symptoms.

The main therapy of these patients is melatonin, combined with behavioral recommendations, where it is important for the patient to have regular meals and activities and physical exercise. Usually the patients received 3-10 mg of melatonin approximately 1 hours before bedtime, and after the rhythm has been stabilized, they receive a daily low dose (0.5 mg) to prevent that the condition comes back.

Jetlag disorder

Jetlag disorder is a result of travelling across several time zones resulting in a mismatch of the internal clock and the clock at the destination local time. The symptoms often come within 1-2 days after travelling. The usual symptoms when a person is suffering from jetlag are sleep disturbances, fatigue, reduced daytime alertness, poor appetite, depressed mood, irritability, and reduced cognitive performance. The jetlag condition is worse when travelling eastwards than when travelling westwards.

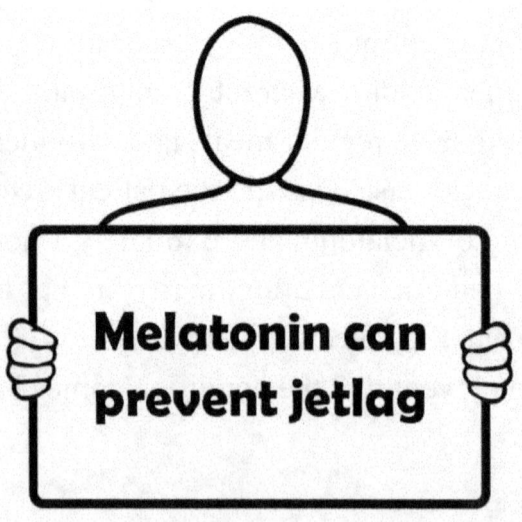

Melatonin can prevent jetlag

There are multiple treatment possibilities for jetlag. The main focus is to get better sleep and improve alertness during the day. There has been focus on the effects of light exposure with avoiding of light at specific times of the day and exposure to light at other times of the day. In treatment of jetlag, melatonin is important. Due to the fact that is has an effect on the circadian system and on sleep one should take 0.5 to10 mg of melatonin in the early evening hours several days before eastwards travel followed by administration at bedtime at the destination. This will reduce the symptoms of jetlag in 50% of individuals with jetlag.

Shift-work

Worldwide it is approximately 15 to 20% of the work force that, in some way is engaged in shift-work. Not all that are engaged in shift-work suffers from shift-work disorder. Among those who are engaged in shift-work, it is approximately 10% that have shift-work disorder. Excessive sleepiness is a common symptom, but also fatigue and mood disorders and decreased libido is seen. There is also an increased risk of substance abuse and alcohol abuse. A lot of co-morbidities are related to shift-work disorder such as risk of weight gain, high blood pressure and heart disease. Finally it has also been shown, that shift-work disorder is correlated with breast- and uterus cancer. Again, there is an effect of a combination of light therapy at specific times, but also if melatonin is taken at bedtime it can improve daytime sleep.

Insomnia

Insomnia is another word for sleeplessness where the person has difficulty to fall asleep or stay asleep as long as he or she wishes. Insomnia can both be acute and chronic. Approximately 5-35% of the population suffers from insomnia. It is known, that the elderly suffers more from insomnia, and also women, people who are less educated or unemployed, medically ill patients, those with depression,

anxiety or has substance
abuse has insomnia.
Most often, patients with
insomnia have fatigue or
reduced motivation,
lower concentration,
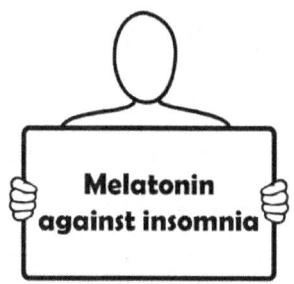
memory disturbances, tendency for depression
and anxiety, headache, intestinal problems or
muscle pain. Melatonin levels in the elderly are
lower than in the younger.

It is known, that treatment with melatonin
results in improved sleep with reduced
symptoms correlated to sleep. There have been
developed different tablets and different
versions of melatonin that have been changed
in the molecular structure and all these have
proven to have an effect on reducing symptoms
related to insomnia. Worldwide, the most often
used indication for melatonin with regards to
treatment of sleep is sleep problems in the
elderly. It has also been shown, that melatonin
can better sleep in patients that are undergoing
some kind of surgery.

MELATONIN AS AN ANTIOXIDANT

As described in the previous chapters melatonin has primarily been investigated in relation to treatment of circadian disorders or sleep disturbances. Within the last 20 to 30 years there has been a tremendous interest in other effects of melatonin. One of the major interests is the antioxidant effect of melatonin. Professor Russel Reiter from Texas University Health Centre has been a pioneer in examining the antioxidant effects of melatonin. When a molecule is described as being an antioxidant it means, that it can block the dangerous effects on cells by reducing the toxicity of so called free radicals. Free radicals are molecules that are highly unstable and which readily react with nearby molecules that are important for cell function and cell maintenance and thus damage cells resulting in death or dysfunction. Another very important aspect of the dangerous effects of free radicals is, that they can damage the DNA within the cell and hereby result in a process, which ultimately can result in cancer.

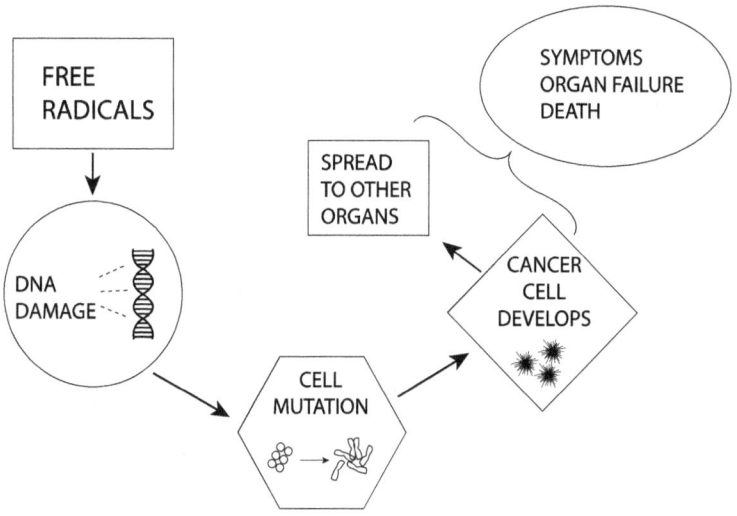

Free radicals can result in cancer through damage to DNA in the cells.

Melatonin is a very strong molecule that can block free radicals. There are a lot of known antioxidants such as vitamin E or beta-carotene. These antioxidants are also important for human function. However, melatonin has been shown to be a stronger antioxidant than these. The mechanisms whereby melatonin acts as an antioxidant is by reducing the highly reactive oxygen molecule that is a central part of a free radical. Thus, melatonin converts the highly toxic oxygen molecule to normal oxygen which is completely without danger for the cells. Another important aspect of melatonin as an antioxidant is, that it starts some other mechanisms in the cells that also functions as antioxidants. This indirect effect is by melatonin activating enzymes that are strong antioxidants. A cell functions like a "mini-factory" where the most active organ using oxygen is the so-called mitochondria. This is a site, where there is a lot of production of these free radicals. Melatonin can stabilize mitochondrial function and hereby also prevent the production of antioxidants and prevent that these mitochondria do not function properly.

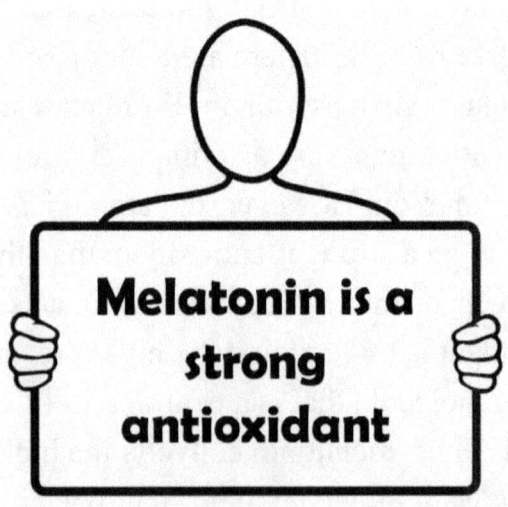

Due to these very important antioxidant effects of melatonin and due to the fact that melatonin can pass through almost any cells in the body because it is soluble in water and in fat, melatonin has many potential effects in diseases where free radicals may be important. It is obvious that oxygen is extremely important for all cells in the body and therefore it is also easy to understand, that free radicals may induce diseases in any organ in the body and finally this leads to the understanding that melatonin may be preventive of disease in many different organs. In the following, some of the most important and interesting effects that melatonin can have as an antioxidant in various serious diseases will be presented.

Melatonin and its antioxidant effects in heart disease

The human heart is an organ, which is highly dependent on oxygen. The heart is pumping out blood in the body 60 to 80 times a minute and therefore is continuously in need of oxygen to function probably. Therefore, the heart is dependent on a blood supply that, if it is reduced, will result in potential lethal consequences. Occlusion of the blood vessels to the heart can occur due to many different reasons including tobacco use, obesity, diabetes, male sex, and due to genetic reasons. Millions of patients worldwide suffer from the potentially lethal consequences of a blood clot or a closure of one or more of these blood vessels. As soon as there is a closed blood vessel to the heart, the patient most often will experience severe chest pain, which if it does not kill the patient, will result in the need for acute medical care. Here the doctors will try to open this blood vessel by removing the reason for the closed blood vessel. This means that there will be some parts of the heart which will be without blood and thus without oxygen for several hours until the blood vessel has been opened. When the blood vessel gets opened due to medical therapy or due to a procedure from a cardiac specialist by introducing a catheter within the blood vessel, the blood vessel opens. This results in a lot of blood with high concentration of oxygen, which goes out to the part of the heart that has been without oxygen for several hours. By intuition this should be a good thing. And it is, however, the high concentration of oxygen to a part of the heart that did not have any oxygen for several hours, results in a phenomenon called ischemia and reperfusion injury. This basically means that there will be generated a lot of these dangerous free radicals, which by themselves can result in cell death and poor function of the heart.

As described in the introduction, melatonin is a very potent antioxidant. There have been numerous animal experiments which in mice, rats, pigs, dogs and other experimental animals have shown, that melatonin can prevent damage to the heart. There are now some trials in humans where it has been shown that melatonin may prevent damage to the heart when there is a high concentration of free radicals. This has gained a great interest around the world and there are now further trials in humans where it is investigated if melatonin given at the time where the closed vessel is opened may reduce the dangerous effects of melatonin. The potential of this highly probable effect are huge and due to its low toxicity melatonin might have a place in the treatment of this large number of patients.

There have been various studies where the melatonin level in the blood has been correlated to the risk of having a heart attack. Studies of patients with so-called unstable and stable angina are interesting in this context. Unstable angina is a condition where there is a high risk of getting a heart attack even when they are not doing any hard exercise, thus the name unstable angina. The patient will have chest pain without any previous activities. In stable angina the patient will experience chest pain due to activities such as physical exercise, going from a hot to a cold environment or after eating a meal. It has been shown that, compared to healthy individuals in the same age and with the same risk factors, a lower level of melatonin in the blood is a risk factor for developing unstable and stable angina.

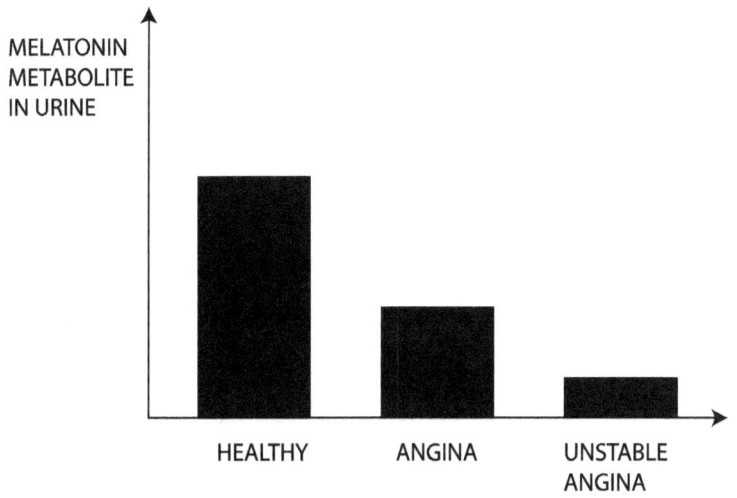

Melatonin protects the heart and the low concentrations are seen in patients with unstable heart disease.

Melatonin as an antioxidant in the brain - melatonin for treatment of stroke

Just as heart attacks due to a closed blood vessel to the heart, one of the other major diseases of the western world is due to closure of blood vessels to the brain. Millions of patients are suffering from this every year and the reason for having an obstructed vessel to the brain resembles the reasons for obstruction of blood vessels to the heart. Thus, it is risk factors such as smoking, diabetes, hypotension and high cholesterol. Just as in the heart, the main focus for the emergency treatment of stroke is to alleviate the symptoms caused by a closed blood vessel to the brain. The underlying disease causing a reduced blood supply to the brain may not always be due to closure of a vessel, but could also be due to other reasons such as brain injury due to trauma, bleeding due to a ruptured vessel or very, very low blood pressure due to another disease. When there is lack of blood and thus oxygen supply to a part of the brain, this results in cellular changes that in turn results in poor cell function and especially also poor function of the important mitochondria, and this results in increased free radical production. The overproduction of free radicals in these mitochondria cannot be neutralized by the antioxidant mechanisms within the cells, and this results in further brain cell damages.

Numerous researchers have shown in

animal experiments, that giving melatonin in relation to low blood supply to a part of the brain, results in very effective prevention of free radical damage and finally a prevention of cell death, resulting in improved brain function. The reason why melatonin is this effective is, that it readily passes through to the cells in the brain and blocks directly the free radicals and improves the function of these important mitochondria. There are no human studies that can support an effect on patients with acute brain disease. It is anticipated, that these investigations will be performed in the near future.

Melatonin in relation to organ transplantation

There are many patients worldwide that due to different reasons are ending up having an organ that do not function. Thanks to the tremendous development in medicine and surgery, it is now possible to transplant organs from one patient to another. A good example of organ transplantations is transplantation of the liver and kidneys. In order to replace an organ, one needs to remove the organ that does not function. All organs in the body have a blood supply and this is interrupted when the sick organ is taken out. Afterwards, when the donor organ is placed inside the patient, the blood supply is re-established. The donor organ has in a variable amount of time been without blood supply. When the blood vessels are attached to the donor organ, the blood supply suddenly increases and this results in a high production of free radicals that induce damage to the cells of the donor organ. Due to the well known antioxidant effects of melatonin, there have been several animal studies, investigating if melatonin could prevent these cell damages and thus prevent the bad function of a new donor organ. Both studies with liver transplantation and kidney transplantation in animals have been performed. These studies show, that melatonin is very effective on preventing free radical damage, and this can both be seen when the cells of the new organ is investigated with a microscope, and when markers of cell damage are examined. Again, there is need of studies in humans to investigate if these effects in animal models can be reproduced. The potential for these patients are great because a considerable portion of these patients either suffer from the consequences of free radical damage or loses their organ due to this free radical damage.

Melatonin for prevention of birth related complications

Luckily the vast majority of births are completely safe and without complications. Knowing which huge changes in body functions that happen both in the mother and in the baby during the birth, it is almost incomprehensible that there are no more complications than actually seen. In the final phases of the birth there are periods of low oxygen supply to the baby due to compression of blood vessels to the placenta. This results in periods of low and high delivery of blood and thus, in periods with low and high concentration of oxygen to the fetus. Reduced oxygen supply to the fetus can also be caused by a condition called preeclampsia, which is a condition, where the mother has high blood pressure. All these effects can in certain cases, result in diseases and complications to the mother and complications to the newborn. Melatonin levels are increased in the end of pregnancy indicating that it is an important substance in the final phase of pregnancy.

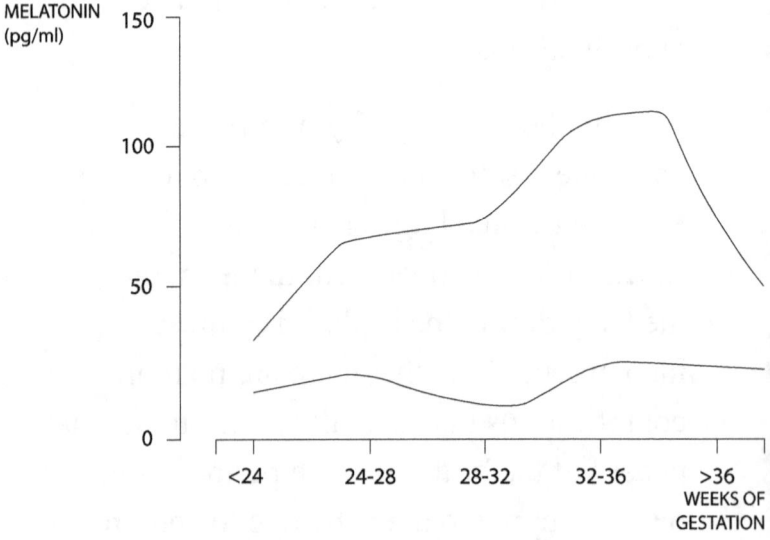

Melatonin concentrations during the night (top line) and day (bottom line) during pregnancy.

There have been performed several studies

investigating if melatonin can have a positive effect in situations, where the blood supply to the placenta and thus the fetus is reduced. Again, the intriguing part of using melatonin within this context is its very low toxicity also in the newborn baby. Due to its chemical properties, melatonin can readily pass through the placenta and to the baby in all phases of pregnancy and delivery. It has been shown, that given melatonin to pregnant rats where the placenta blood flow has been stopped for a period resembling what is happening during preeclampsia or during birth, results in improved growth of the fetus within the uterus and also can result in reduced damage to the newborn. Again, this has tremendous importance in humans if melatonin could be given to women with high risk of damage to the fetus, due to pregnancy related complications or due to complications during the birth process.

MELATONIN AND THE IMMUNE SYSTEM

A well functioning immune system is of extreme importance in the daily living of living organisms. If there is a severe malfunction of the immune system for a longer period this will almost inevitably result in death due to infection. The human organism is constantly under attack of potentially harmful exposures due to bacteria, viruses or environmental pollutions. The immune system is active every second of the day and is clearing and combatting these external threats. Various diseases can result in either acute or chronic immune dysfunction. Another aspect of diseases in the immune system is when there is a so-called autoimmune disease resulting in attack of tissues in the body because the immune system is overactive. One of the most known diseases that can cause severe immune dysfunction due to infection is a virus infection by the HIV virus. There are many chronic autoimmune diseases and one of the most known are rheumatoid arthritis affecting the joints.

In the 1970'ies the first studies examining lack of melatonin was made in animal experiments. Cells of the immune system are found in every organ of the body and also found in specific organs such as lymph nodes, spleen and the thymus and in high concentration in the intestines. These immune active cells are the first line of defense. Researchers investigated whether the surgical removal of the pineal gland where a major part of the melatonin production is, would result in immune dysfunction. The surgical removal of the pineal

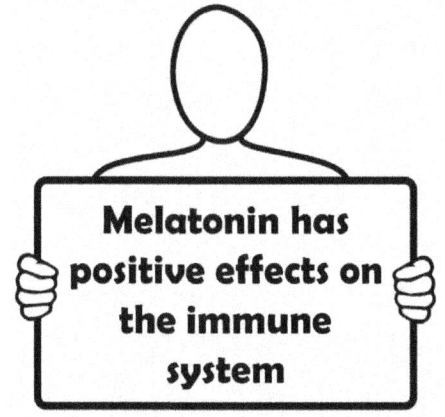

Melatonin has positive effects on the immune system

gland results in an abolished melatonin secretion to the blood and this secondarily resulted in a severe lack of immune cells in the blood and in the spleen and also reduction of the size of the lymph nodes. Thus, the immune organs were reduced in size and function. This has been shown in animal experiments to result in loss of ability to prevent the damaging effects by dangerous bacteria's. Immune cells are producing molecules called cytokines, which are important for the immune response. If an animal has its pineal gland removed, it results in a reduced amount of cytokines indicating reduced immune function. When melatonin is given to the animals that do not have a pineal gland because of surgical removal, it actually results in normalization of the production of the cytokines and this is a strong proof of the effect of melatonin on immune function. A further indication of the effects of melatonin on the immune system is based on investigations of animals with a long period of biological night. Here, it is shown that if the daytime period is short and the night period is long resulting in higher melatonin concentrations during the night, this results in improved immune function compared with the opposite situation with a long daytime period and short nighttime period.

The above-mentioned studies are all focusing on the effect of normal or no presence of melatonin. There have also been studies where melatonin administration has been examined in different situation where the immune system is under a large stress. Even when the immune system is not under a large stress, treatment with melatonin results in larger immune active organs. During infection where it is extremely important that the immune system is functioning well it has been shown that melatonin can reduce the deleterious effects of infections. In many different studies in animals the treatment with melatonin, when the animals are exposed to a severe infection, results in improved immune function and increased survival. There have also been human studies investigating the relationship between melatonin and the immune system.

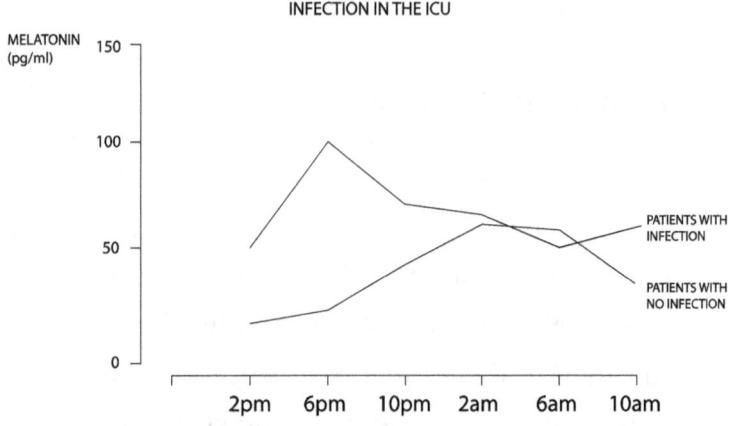

Melatonin plays a role during severe diseases. Different levels are seen in patients with and without infection indicating that melatonin may be important for a patient to overcome an infection.

It has been shown in healthy young people, that there is a circadian difference in the immune system depending on time of day. In experimental studies in humans, who received a mild infection due to injection of bacteria into the blood, it was shown that there was a significant difference between the response when the bacteria are injected in the daytime where there is no melatonin compared with the nighttime where there is a high melatonin concentration. In humans, who has an HIV infection it has been shown that the function of immune cells are corresponding to the level of melatonin in the blood. All these studies are indicating that melatonin is important for immune related functions in the human. Due to all these proofs of a positive effect of melatonin there have also been clinical studies where melatonin has been given to humans during infection. This has been done in newborns with blood infections where it was shown that melatonin administration in high concentrations actually resulted in improved survival in the newborns who received melatonin compared with newborns who did not get treatment with melatonin. Different studies are performed at the moment around the world, examining if these results can be reproduced.

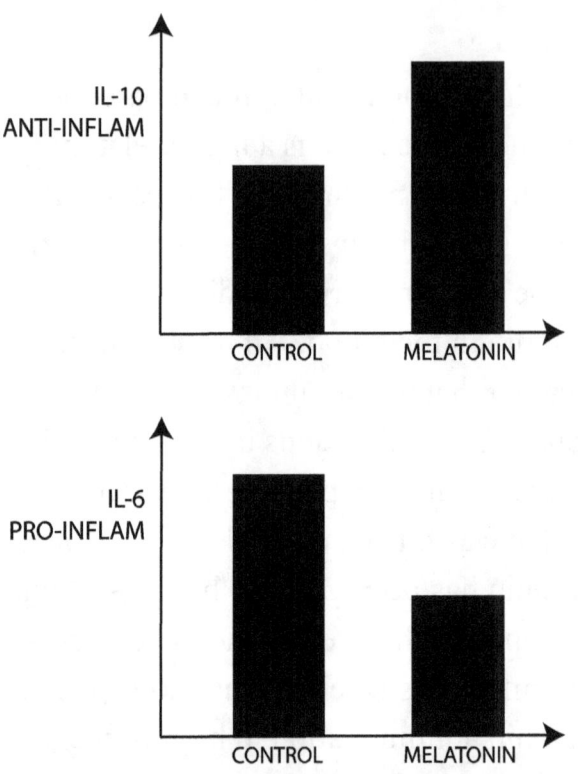

IL-10 is a so-called anti-inflammatory cytokine and IL-6 on the contrary promotes inflammation. In study subjects where inflammation is started by giving a certain substance promoting inflammation it can be seen that treatment with melatonin results in reduced inflammation by increasing the IL-10 and reducing the IL-6.

A healthy immune system is not only important when there are infections. A healthy immune system is also extremely important in the combat against cancer. As indicated in the above, melatonin administration increased the size of immune organs and improved the function of immune cells. Several studies in humans with different cancers have shown that melatonin by itself but especially when combined with the so-called cytokines. This ultimately can result in improved treatment of patients with cancer.

CLINICAL EFFECTS OF MELATONIN

Melatonin is primarily secreted from the pineal gland and regulated by the environmental light and dark circle. It is primarily involved in sleep regulation and regulation of other cyclical body activities. In both human and animals it is primarily regulating the clock and the calendar, i.e. it regulates "time of day" and "time of year", but melatonin has also many other diverse functions in the body which is not depending directly on the secretion of melatonin from the pineal gland but depends on local production of melatonin in different organs and tissues throughout the body. Examples of these are production of melatonin in the intestines, in the bone marrow, in white blood cells and in the skin. The production in these organs is not only concerned with cyclical function of the cells, but also preventive measures due to the antioxidant effect of melatonin. Due to these factors melatonin has been investigated in many different disease conditions. At the moment there are many animal experiments that show some important potential effects of this hormone. Within the last 5-10 years there have been an increasing number of clinical studies that suggests that melatonin may have a place for treatment of various diseases and conditions. Within the next section of this chapter, we will run through some of the major conditions/diseases, where melatonin has been investigated and potentially will have an effect for treatment of humans.

Heart disease

In a previous chapter regarding the antioxidant effect of melatonin in acute heart attack it was described, that melatonin has strong antioxidant effects when the heart is suffering due to closure of the blood vessels that provide blood to the working heart. In addition to this preventive effect in acute heart disease, melatonin also has a preventive effect on atherosclerosis which is calcification of the blood vessels and it has also been shown to be effective in treating increased blood pressure and to have an effect on the prevention of the side effects on the heart by various drugs which are used to treat cancer or to treat patients that have received an organ transplantation.

The antioxidant effect of melatonin in heart attack has been described in previous chapters. In the following, the effects of melatonin in other heart conditions will be described.

Atherosclerosis

Atherosclerosis is a chronic disease in the blood vessels where oxidative stress and inflammation are major factors in the development. High concentrations of cholesterol in the blood, seems to be important in the development of atherosclerosis.

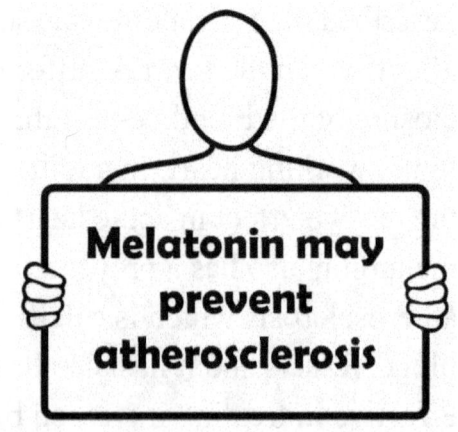

One of the important cholesterol molecules that

are important in this context is the low so-called low density lipoproteins (LDL). When this molecule is oxidized, it is an important factor in the development of atherosclerosis. It has been shown in laboratory studies, that melatonin and its metabolites may reduce the oxidization of LDL and thus prevent atherosclerosis.

Melatonin may also reduce other cholesterols in the blood leading to preventive effects. This effect on the blood lipids is also induced by the activation by other antioxidant enzymes by melatonin. This has been shown in animal experiments where weeks of treatment with melatonin reduced atherosclerosis. As described previously, melatonin also has an effect in the immune system. The inflammation process, which is a situation where the immune system is active, is central for development of atherosclerosis. It has been shown, that the anti-inflammatory effect of melatonin may again reduce atherosclerosis.

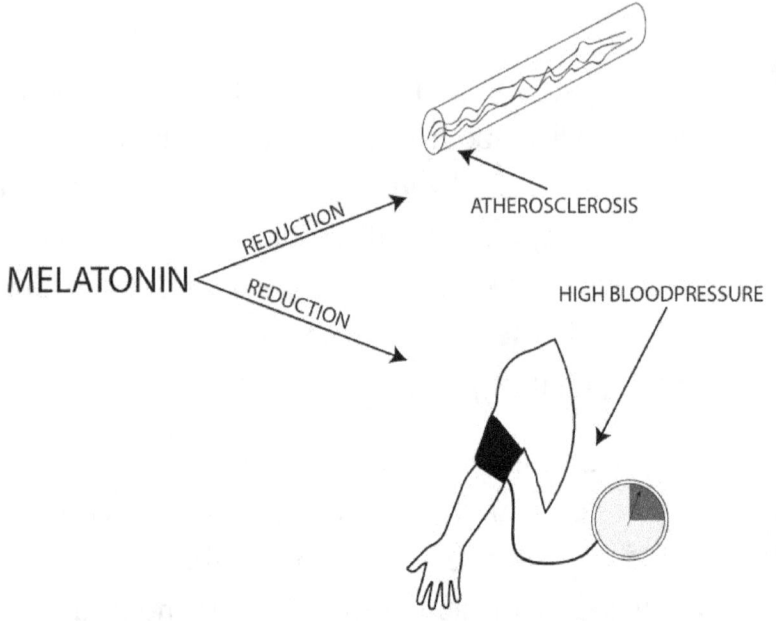

Melatonin can have very positive effects in heart disease by both lowering the blood pressure and by reducing atherosclerosis (calcification in the major blood vessels).

Melatonin and high blood pressure

Millions of patients are suffering from high blood pressure, and this is a condition that can result in heart attack, stroke, kidney problems and other serious diseases. It has been proposed by several researchers that melatonin may have a positive effect on the treatment of high blood pressure, because it will normalize the variation of blood pressure that is important for body functions. Thus, the best situation is a blood pressure that rises in the daytime where there is bodily activities and falls during the night, where the person is laying down, sleeping and does not need a high blood pressure to maintain body functions. Many patients with high blood pressure are not able to regulate their blood pressure during the night and are continuously in a high blood pressure at these hours. This is an important risk factor, for development of diseases that are associated with high blood pressure. Melatonin has been supposed to reduce the blood pressure by giving signals to the brain that it is night and therefore, when it is taken in the evening hours, it will cause a healthy reduction in blood pressure in the night time hours. There have been several studies in patients with high blood pressure and these are showing, that melatonin has a significant effect on lowering blood pressure both during the day and during the night.

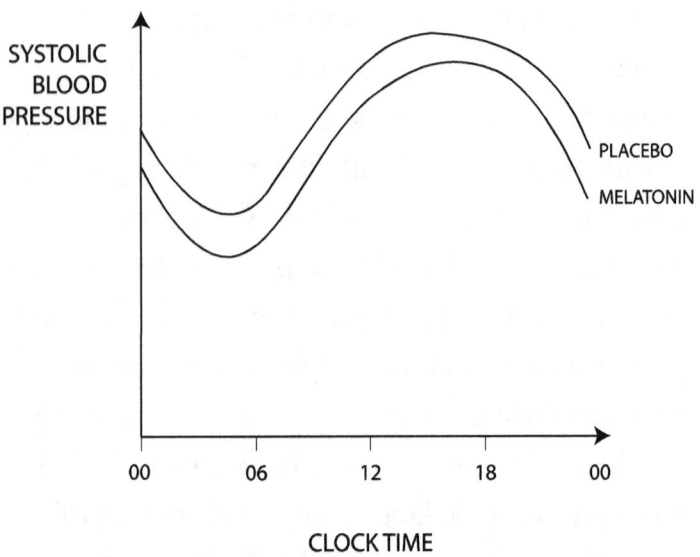

Melatonin results in lowering of the blood pressure compared with placebo.

This was also shown in patients with other risk factors such as diabetes. Due to its low toxicity, it is certainly a drug that should be considered in the treatment of high blood pressure. This may be either as a stand-alone treatment or in addition to other drugs that also has an effect on the blood pressure. In addition to its effect on the brain, the positive effects of melatonin treatment may also be connected to its direct effect in the

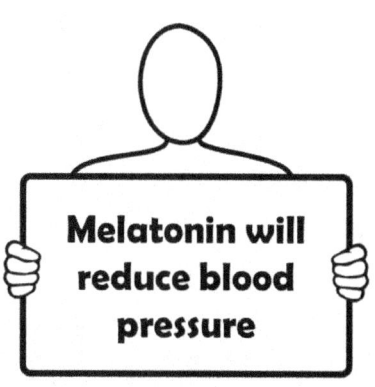

heart muscle and in the very small blood vessels in the organs. It is believed, that these effects in patients with high blood pressure may be due to its antioxidant effect.

The doses that have been shown to be effective in the treatment of women with high blood pressure or patients with diabetes have been in the range of 2-3 mg of melatonin in the evening.

Melatonin for prevention of side effects of other drugs

There have been tremendous developments of treatment of cancer with development of many drugs that can kill the cancer cells and ultimately cure the patient due to these effects. As it is generally known, most of these drugs have side effects because they are also affecting normal cells in the body. Especially certain chemotherapeutics such as cisplatine, bleomycine, epirobicine or doxorubicine are known to induce oxidative stress in addition or as a part of their effects on cancer cells. Another drug, which is uses in various diseases, is cyclosporine A that reduces the function of the immune system. It is therefore used in different conditions where this is wanted, such as autoimmune disease or in patients that have received a donor organ.

Patients that receive the above-mentioned drugs may suffer from side effects on the heart and ultimately some patients actually die because of the chemotherapeutic treatment. Due to this knowledge, there has been major focus on trying to prevent the side effects of these drugs in humans. There have been numerous studies on animals treated with chemotherapeutics or drugs such as cyclosporine and these studies have shown some encouraging results. Thus, it has been shown that the negative effects on the heart cells due to the oxidative stress that is produced by chemotherapeutics can be blocked completely by giving melatonin. These effects have been shown in different animal species and there is a need of further studies in humans in order to show if the same effects can be reproduced and thus if it can benefit some of these patients that are in high risk. Again, it is important to underline, the low toxicity of melatonin and to emphasize that many patients that receive chemotherapeutics are elderly and thus are in a higher risk of having other conditions that also effects the heart negatively such as diabetes, high blood pressure or atherosclerosis.

Melatonin for treatment of cancer

After showing that nurses that are working more than 4-5 shifts during the night in one month are increased risk of having breast cancer and colorectal cancer there have been a lot of focus on this. The mechanism involved is believed to be due to light exposure in the night, resulting in no melatonin increase during the night and thus no antioxidant effect of melatonin, in more than 4 to 5 nights in a month. In order to examine the mechanisms underlying this, there have been some interesting experiments in laboratory cancer research that have supported, that melatonin may have a direct cancer preventive effect. In a study of cancer in animals, the blood from women that were exposed to light during the night and blood from women that was not exposed to light during the night were injected into animals with cancer.

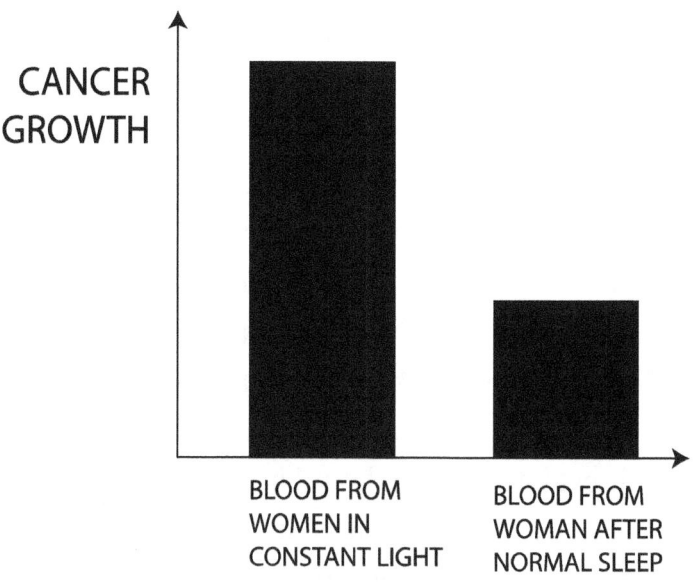

CANCER
GROWTH

BLOOD FROM
WOMEN IN
CONSTANT LIGHT

BLOOD FROM
WOMAN AFTER
NORMAL SLEEP

The blood from women that were exposed to light during the night resulted in increased cancer growth when injected into animals with cancer.

The study showed that the cancer cells that were exposed to blood from the women with high melatonin concentration (patients that were not exposed to light) resulted in a significant reduction in tumor size. Based on this, there have also been a lot of other studies, also in patients where the effects of melatonin in the treatment of cancer have been examined.

Recently, clinical trials using melatonin as an add-on to the other chemotherapeutic agents in patients with advanced cancer were made. A meta-analysis (a scientific method to report all clinical trials in a single combined analysis) showed, that melatonin treatment for patients with so-called solid cancers resulted in dramatic effects. The patients in the eight studies that were examined were patients with metastatic lung, breast, intestinal, and brain cancers. All these patients were in active treatment with other chemotherapeutic regimens and the studies were based on adding melatonin or placebo in addition to their treatment. The meta-analysis showed, that melatonin improved complete and partial remission which means that the size of tumors in the patients was significantly reduced. In addition it also was shown, that the one-year survival rate was higher in the patients treated with melatonin compared with the placebo group.

Another encouraging result was the effect on prevention of toxic reactions to chemotherapy. It showed, that melatonin treatment resulted in reduced fatigue and also significantly reduced toxic reactions in the brain and also had a pronounced effect on the negative effects on blood cells (platelets). Finally, the analysis showed that there were no severe adverse events. Many of the studies in this meta-analysis has been made by a single author group, and it is very important that additional studies are performed in order to reproduce these results, and thereby introduce this treatment to patients with cancer. An important reason why these studies

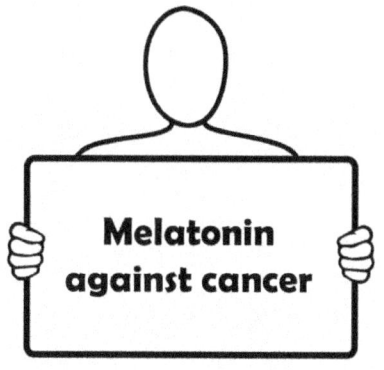

are not performed is that there is no patent for melatonin, and this means that the multi-national drug companies are not interested in supporting scientists to do these trials. It is the hope of the authors to that there will be governmental support for these kinds of trials, so these potentially very important implications of melatonin treatment for cancer can be confirmed. There are certainly a lot of studies in animals that are showing that it is not merely in situations where there are metastatic cancer (cancer that has spread to other organs than the primary organ where the cancer originated), but also effects in primary tumors. This has been shown in breast cancer, in uterus cancer, ovarian cancer, prostate cancer, liver cancer, skin cancer, and colorectal cancer.

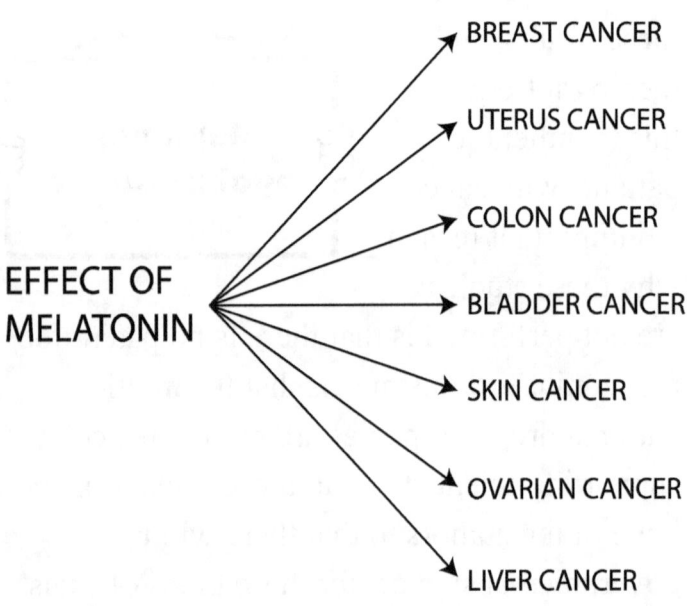

EFFECT OF
MELATONIN

BREAST CANCER

UTERUS CANCER

COLON CANCER

BLADDER CANCER

SKIN CANCER

OVARIAN CANCER

LIVER CANCER

Melatonin for treatment of depression

In order to understand the effect of melatonin in depression it is important to remember the effect of melatonin for sleep problems. Usually, the treatment of sleeplessness is by giving patients a so-called sleeping pill which. Until recently, the drugs that have been used have been in the benzodiazepine drug group. These substances have been shown to be effective in inducing and maintaining sleep. However, there are also some serious side effects to these drugs. The major concern in treatment with benzodiazepines is, that these drugs induce tolerance, even after shorter period of treatments. The sleep that is induced by benzodiazepines is also not "healthy sleep". Benzodiazepines results in change of the sleep architecture and also result in hang-over effects in the morning resulting in fatigue and in the elderly that ultimately can result in accidents due to these effects. Melatonin with its prominent hypnotic effect and its effect on stabilizing circadian rhythms is an obvious drug for the treatment of insomnia, and is now recommended by different scientific societies for treatment of sleeplessness in the elderly patients over 55 years of age. There are many millions of patients around the world that are suffering from sleeplessness, and the drug companies have shown a great interest in developing drugs that have an effect as melatonin. Thus, there has been development of several melatonin analogues that has been approved by different medical authorities around the World.

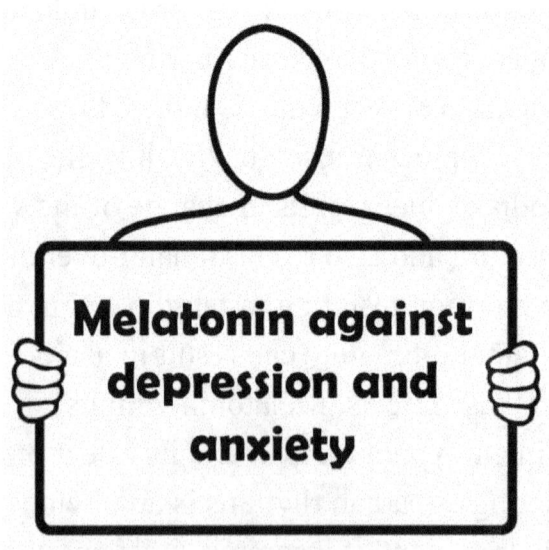

Sleeplessness or insomnia is a central part of being depressed. Insomnia is actually a part of the diagnostic criteria for depressive disorder. There have been different medical studies on patients with depression that show, that melatonin is effective in inducing sleep in patients with depression, but in addition, also has an effect on treating depression. Thus, several studies of melatonin analogues has shown these anti-depressive effects and actually due to their lower side-effects and due to their pronounced effect on sleep problems, there have been shown to be better than the usual anti-depressive drugs. One of these anti-depressants are called agomelatin, and this has been extensively studied. The difference between melatonin and agomelatin is that agomelatin has effects on melatonin receptors, but in addition, also an effect on the serotonin-system that are central for treatment of depression. However, recent studies have shown that it is not necessary for a drug to have an effect on the serotonin-system in order to be antidepressant. A proof of this is studies where melatonin treatment for depression after surgery for breast cancer in women, has been shown to prevent depressive symptoms and improve sleep compared with placebo. Also one of the analogues to melatonin, that is only affecting melatonin receptors and not the serotonergic system, has in clinical trials shown to have anti-depressant effects in patients with depression. The side effects of the newly developed melatonin-like drugs are not investigated in details and there are concerns, that some of these drugs may affect treatment with other drugs and might result in side effects due to this. Therefore, it seems like it is not necessary to use the commercial melatonin analogues. Until further data has been shown, it seems like that pure melatonin treatment might be sufficient for treating and preventing depression. As described, a special focus group is the large group of women treated for breast cancer, where treatment with melatonin compared with placebo, has been shown to improve sleep and prevent depressive symptoms.

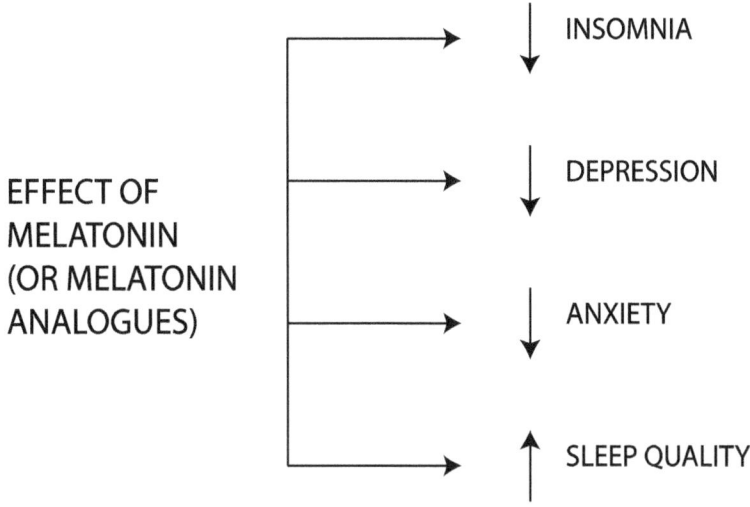

Various important effects of melatonin or its analogues in persons with sleep problems and psychiatric complaints.

Melatonin for treatment of diabetes

In 2013, the results from a major study from Harvard showed that there is a tight connection between the concentration of melatonin and development of type-2 diabetes. It was shown, that lower concentrations of melatonin is associated with the development of diabetes. Thus, the hypothesis that melatonin might have a protective effect in the development of diabetes is very likely.

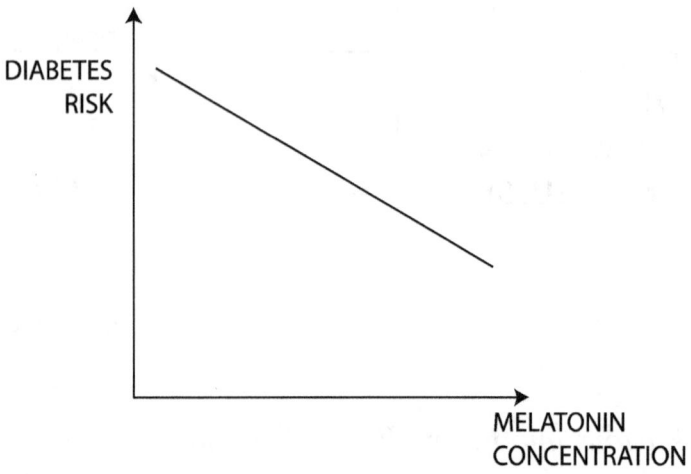

The risk of having diabetes is reduced if the concentration of melatonin is high in the person.

There have been different trials that have shown similar effects in patients with various complications or with various aspects of type-2 diabetes. It has been shown, that when patients have a low concentration of melatonin they are more likely to have diabetes or to develop diabetes. This hypothesis is strengthened by the observation in shift-workers or in persons with shorter sleep duration compared with longer sleep duration. It has been shown, that if one are sleeping less than 5 hours/night they have a higher likelihood to develop diabetes compared with sleeping 7 hours/night.

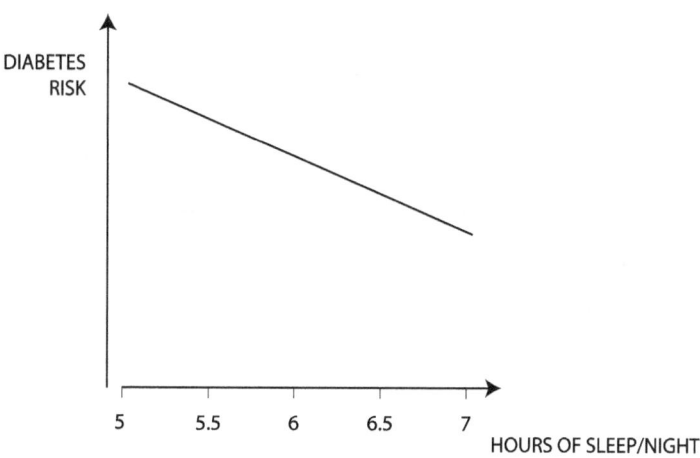

People sleeping less than 5 hours/night have a higher likelihood of developing diabetes compared with sleeping 7 hours/night.

This is also shown in patients that snore. Patients snoring have a much higher risk of developing type-2 diabetes compared with those that do not snore. There are only a limited number of studies comparing melatonin with placebo for

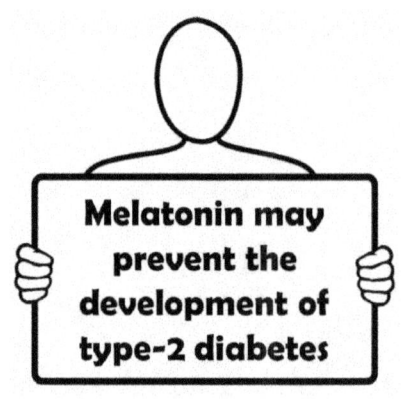

Melatonin may prevent the development of type-2 diabetes

treatment of diabetes. These preliminary studies suggest that melatonin treatment may reduce high levels of sugar in the blood, may reduce blood lipids and actually may also reduce obesity. It is particularly the abdominal obesity i.e. fat around the organs that is particularly dangerous and that actually may be reduced mostly by melatonin treatment. It will be very interesting in the future to see the results from clinical trials that are ongoing these years and to see if melatonin treatment will have an effect in the treatment of diabetes and the metabolic syndrome.

Melatonin for treatment of epilepsy

Epilepsy is a very common disease affecting almost 1% of the population. Due to this high occurrence of this disease, there have been a tremendous focus and development of drugs for treatment of epilepsy. In spite of this, almost 1/3 of patients with epilepsy cannot have their seizures prevented by the current medical treatment possibilities. Many patients with epilepsy has a day and night difference in the occurrence of their seizures and it has been hypothesized, that melatonin may have an effect in seizure prevention. Melatonin has an effect on some of the receptors in the brain that is central for developing seizures in patients with epilepsy. It has been, primarily in children, been shown that there is a lower melatonin concentration in the blood in children with seizures compared with those that do not have seizures. This is not a proof of causality. However, it has been shown, that melatonin effects the receptors (GABA-receptors) in the brain that are central for seizure development and many animal studies has actually shown melatonin to be effective in prevention of seizures. There has been one human randomized clinical trial that have shown an effect in seizure prevention. However, this was not possible to show in two other studies. Thus, it is not possible to conclude if melatonin may be a drug that can be used in seizure treatment and this should be investigated further, in the future.

Melatonin for treatment of pain

Pain is involved in the vast majority of diseases that we know of, at one time or the other. Pain is almost an inevitable part of surgery. Millions of patients receive surgical procedures for many different diseases and conditions. A central part in the development of pain is tissue damage, resulting in signals to the brain that something wrong is going on. The mechanism underlying pain is local changes that occur in the skin or in the organs when the surgeon operates. It is both the changes locally but also the processing of the brain that is central for the pain experience. There is also numerous chronic pain conditions with pain in the muscular skeletal system as one of the most frequent causes.

Melatonin has been investigated both in acute and chronic pain conditions. The most research that has been made both in animals and in humans is in the setting of acute pain. The mechanism of melatonin in preventing acute pain is believed to be due to its antioxidant and anti-inflammatory effects and due to the effect on the nerve system, where the pain impulse is transmitted to the brain. Anxiety, that is a central part of a patient's response to a situation where there will be pain, or a situation where the patient is anticipating discomfort due to surgery, is an important issue. Thus, many studies investigating pain has also investigated the effects on anxiety. In women undergoing surgery for a gynecological disease it has been shown that melatonin is effective in reducing pain after surgery, but also been shown to be effective in preventing anxiety. One of the most well investigated areas for melatonin is its effects on reducing anxiety before surgery. Treatment with 1-10 mg of melatonin on the night before surgery and 1-2 hours immediately before surgery has been shown to be very effective. The same doses have also been shown to reduce the dose of other drugs for pain treatment and by this, melatonin can reduce the potential serious side effects of these drugs (such as opioids). Melatonin has therefore been incorporated in some departments around the World for treatment of pain related to surgery. Ongoing studies will be examining if the effectiveness of melatonin for pain treatment can be expanded to other areas of acute pain.

For chronic pain conditions, there are also human studies that are showing an effect of melatonin. Some of these chronic pain conditions are fibromyalgia, irritable bowel syndrome and migraine. Fibromyalgia is a condition where patients have muscular pain and difficulty sleeping and it is primarily women that suffer from this disease. The prevalence of this condition is about 2-5% in the Western World. Many of these women are also suffering from depressive disorder. The hypothesis that melatonin might have an effect in these women has been based on the known analgesic effects of melatonin, but also based on the finding, that patients with fibromyalgia has lower melatonin concentrations in blood. Melatonin treatment for women with fibromyalgia (3 mg orally for 4 weeks, half an hour before sleeping time) resulted in improved sleep and reduced muscular pain. An effect on muscular stiffness and depression has also been shown in another study.

Irritable bowel syndrome is a painful condition in the intestines. Again, it has been shown, that patients with irritable bowel syndrome has lower levels of melatonin in the blood compared with healthy volunteers. In these patients, where pain was a very central part of the condition, melatonin treatment with 3 mg of oral melatonin resulted in significantly lower intestinal pain. The overall improvement in their symptoms related to irritable bowel syndrome was also better, after melatonin treatment.

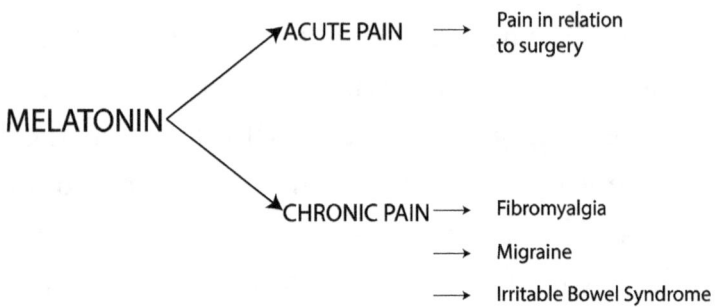

Melatonin has been shown to reduce pain in both acute and chronic pain conditions.

Migraine is a common condition in the Western World. Patients with migraine have lower concentration in melatonin in the blood compared with healthy controls. In a trial of patients with migraine, they received 3 mg of melatonin half an hour before bedtime and in these patients it was shown, that melatonin treatment reduced the frequency of headaches, the severity of headaches and the duration. A positive thing was also, that the patients reduced their intake of other painkillers. Thus, melatonin was believed to have a preventive effect in migraine.

Melatonin for treatment of gastrointestinal disease

A common mechanism in the development of ulcers in the stomach or in the development of colitis, which is an inflammatory disease in the large intestine, is the occurrence of oxidative stress. In patients with reflux-disease or ulcer disease in the stomach, there is a lower concentration of melatonin compared with healthy volunteers. In addition it has been shown, that 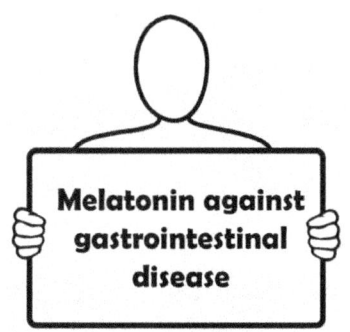 melatonin treatment results in a protection of the lining in the stomach with, a higher production of mucous and protective substances (bicarbonate). This results in a protection of the stomach wall. In patients with reflux-disease, or in patients with ulcers in the stomach, melatonin treatment has been shown to have clinical effects.

The development of symptoms in relation to colitis (bleeding, pain and diarrhea) is probably also related to inflammation and oxidative stress. In patients with colitis it has been shown, that adding melatonin (5 mg at bedtime) compared with placebo results in significantly improved overall symptoms through the 12 months treatment period. The effects of melatonin could also be seen in blood samples, showing less bleeding and less infection in the melatonin group compared with the placebo group.

Further clinical trials will show, if this effect is reproducible and can be added in the treatment of this large group of patients with these serious symptoms.

Melatonin for prevention and treatment of osteoporosis

Osteoporosis is a condition characterized by weakening of the bones and is primarily seen in the elderly and in women. Experimental studies have investigated the association of melatonin and bone strength. In animals, when the pineal gland was removed, it resulted in weakening of the bones. This association with lower melatonin levels and osteoporosis has also been investigated in women. Again, as in other chronic conditions, there are related symptoms due to the chronic pain that can be seen in these patients. In a treatment of women with osteoporosis given 3 mg of melatonin or placebo for 6 months, no effect on the bones could be seen, but there were an improvement of physical symptoms related to osteoporosis in the melatonin group. Further studies should be made before any conclusions can be made in this patient-group.

MELATONIN AGAINST SUN-INDUCED EFFECTS

Sunburn will cause both erythema as well as serious cell damages leading to skin cancer in some individuals. If melatonin is supplied on the skin with e.g. a cream as a carrier, then it will very effectively protect against UVR-induced erythema in humans if applied before the UVR-exposure. This has been shown in several clinical studies, and there seems to be a dose-response effect meaning that the higher the dose, the better the protection against UVR-induced erythema.

Possible side effects

There is, however, a risk of systemic absorption of melatonin through the skin with such a topical application and there may therefore be a risk of slight sedative side effects when used in high concentrations and on larger body areas. This has not been shown in humans, but there is a plausible risk when applying large doses to large skin areas for sun protection. Studies are therefore needed to find the effective dose with the least possible concentration in order to give sun protection at the same time without side effects.

Melatonin against sun-induced skin cancer

Numerous experimental studies have shown, that melatonin on the skin will protect against UVB-induced cell damages that could lead to the development of cancer. This protection is mediated through various mechanisms, and the most important mechanism is probably the ability of melatonin to remove active free oxygen radicals produced by the sun exposure. This protective effect against skin cancer has only been shown in animal studies, and in humans we still need conclusive data to argue for a protective effect against sun induced skin cancers. However, all experimental data point in the same direction and that is a significant protection against the mechanisms ultimately leading to skin cancer.

Melatonin against sunburn

Another mechanism for the protection of melatonin especially against UVR-induced erythema may be the anti-inflammatory effects of melatonin. Thus, the erythema induced by the sun exposure may partly be explained by local inflammation and this can be counteracted by topical administration of melatonin applied before sun exposure. It is unknown, whether melatonin in effective concentrations can be applied to red and sore skin as seen after sunburn. In this situation, there is significant local inflammation in the skin with erythema and pain and it is possible that

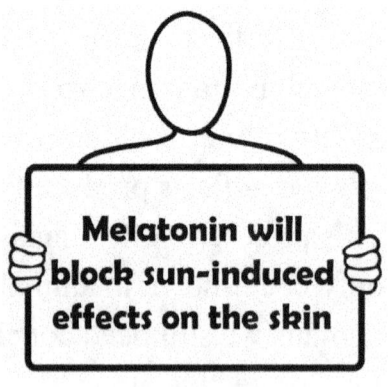

melatonin in the correct dose will also help in this situation. The data for this, however, are not available at the moment. Likewise, it could be hypothesized that taking melatonin tablets in the evening before going to bed after a day with sun exposure potentially could protect against some of the skin cell damages caused by the UVR. Again, however, this has not been studied in humans, but the very effective anti-inflammatory as well oxygen-radical-scavenging effect of melatonin would also be active when taking melatonin as a tablet in the evening. It would therefore be natural to expect some kind of repair mechanisms during the night after sunburn and when taking oral melatonin after the sun exposure.

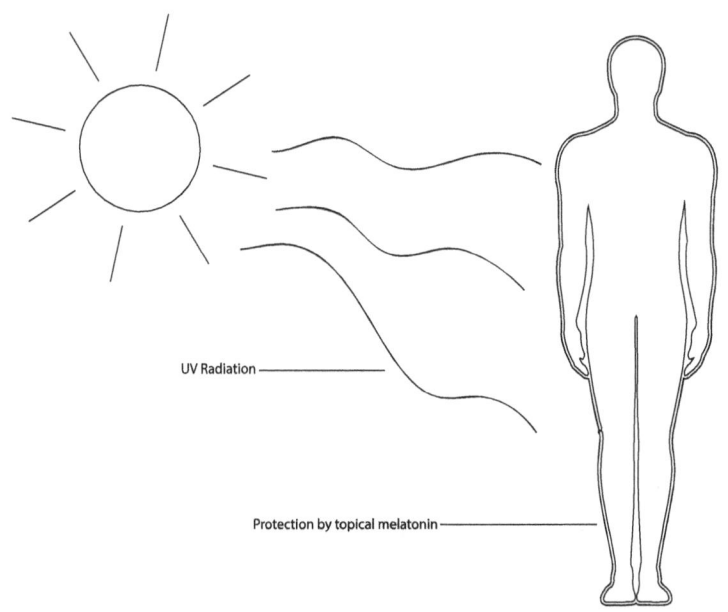

UV Radiation

Protection by topical melatonin

Special patient groups at high risk

Certain patient groups have increased risk of developing skin cancer and that include patients taking immunosuppressive medicine for various clinical conditions and patients with actinic keratosis. These patients have a significantly increased risk of developing non-melanoma skin cancer and the risk is increased with sun exposure. For these patients it would be especially relevant to be able to prevent the cell lesions caused by sun exposure and therefore topical melatonin for these patients seems justified. We do still need, however, dose-finding studies and information about toxicity when applying very high doses of melatonin to the skin with subsequent systemic absorption. Nevertheless, the only clinically relevant side effect that could be expected would be in some patients a slight sedative effect which is the only relevant side-effect that has been found in high dose melatonin given to humans. We therefore with great interest await clinical data in this highly relevant area.

MELATONIN IN WARFARE, NUCLEAR DISASTERS AND OTHER RADIATION INJURIES

Sulfur mustard

Sulfur mustard commonly known as mustard gas is a chemical warfare agent that has also recently been used against the civilian populations in e.g. Syria and Iraq. It is colorless and almost impossible to discover until it is too late. It produces terrible injuries with formation of large blisters on the skin and in the lungs (see picture). The mechanism of injury in sulfur mustard toxicity is primarily caused by oxidative stress and it is therefore natural to think about strong anti-oxidants as possible treatment agents against sulfur mustard toxicity.

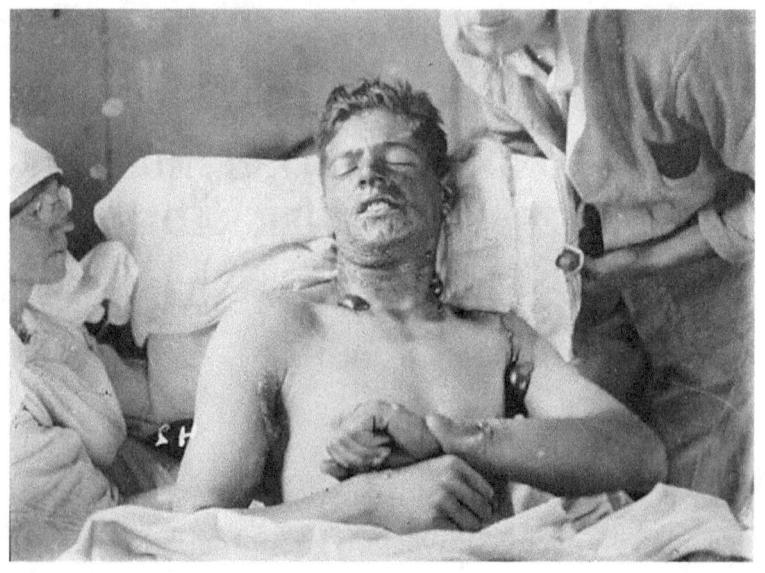

Blisters on neck and arms after exposure to sulfur mustard.

There is currently no good treatment available worldwide. The damage induced by sulfur mustard contains several mechanisms at a molecular level resulting in damage to cell DNA and thereby cell death. Recent studies in rats and in pigs have shown very interesting results where melatonin could counteract the effects of sulfur mustard intoxication. In rats the melatonin was given as injections and it could be shown after sulfur mustard intoxication in these rats that the cell damage was significantly decreased, and melatonin was therefore a protective compound in reducing sulfur mustard toxicity. In pigs it has been shown that applying melatonin as a cream formulation on the skin, the skin damaging effects of sulfur mustard could be significantly reduced.

Therefore, melatonin may prove to be the only current treatment option to counteract deleterious effects of sulfur mustard in chemical warfare. It has to our knowledge not been used in humans yet for this purpose but it would be obvious to provide high-dose melatonin for soldiers engaged in war activities in countries where the use of sulfur mustard as a chemical weapon could be anticipated. As soon as the presence of sulfur mustard is discovered, the soldiers (and of course also the civilian population) could take high dose melatonin as tablets or cream in order to prevent or reduce the toxic effects of sulfur mustard. Melatonin is cheap and absolutely non-toxic so it would be natural to include that in the preventive medical kit for soldiers, and it could be made available for the civilian population as well.

Melatonin in nuclear disasters

The recent nuclear accident at the Fukushima Daiichi Nuclear Power Plant in Japan in 2011 raised the awareness of the need for protective agents against ionizing radiation from nuclear accidents. It has been shown in numerous experimental studies that the deleterious effects of whole body eradiation (as in nuclear accidents) can be somewhat counteracted by the injection of high-dose melatonin. Thus, melatonin has been shown to prevent the death of animals given a small dose of ironizing radiation, and in humans melatonin has been shown to reduce effectively the molecular and cellular damages from ironizing radiation.

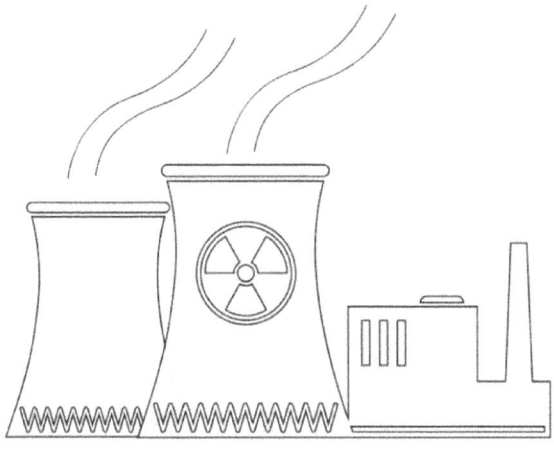

The mechanism of action of melatonin against radiation injuries is primarily its ability to scavenge free oxygen radicals that are produced by the radiation. The effects of melatonin against radiation injury are remarkable and very effective and this held together with the non-toxicity of melatonin as well as the extremely low price makes melatonin an obvious drug against

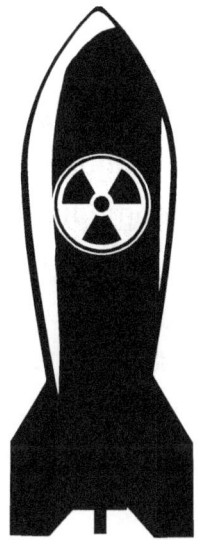

radiation injuries in nuclear disasters. This includes of course disasters at nuclear power plants like the recent one in Japan as well as the effects of radiation injuries caused by "dirty bombs" if used in terrorist attacks.

The side effects of melatonin are negligible or non-existent, and in fact it has not been possible to find a lethal dose in animal experiments. Melatonin has been shown to be superior to other compounds against radiation injuries in numerous experimental studies. Melatonin can be given orally whereas other compounds have to be administered intravenously, and melatonin has very long shelf-life at room temperature

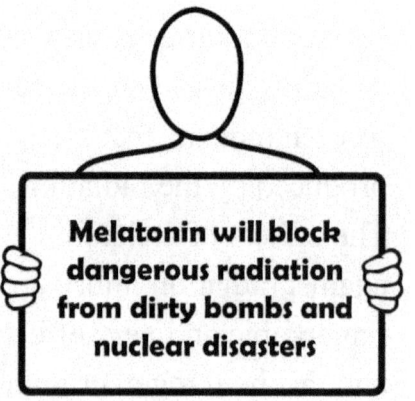

Melatonin will block dangerous radiation from dirty bombs and nuclear disasters

meaning that it can be carried as tablets for a very long time and still be effective when taken orally.

Therefore, the most effective as well as the most practical way to protect people against radiation injury from nuclear accidents or "dirty bombs" would be by ingestion of high-dose oral melatonin.

Melatonin as a radio-protector in clinical oncology

The mechanisms for ionizing radiation damage are both direct and indirect where the indirect effects result from the interaction with water molecules producing highly reactive free radicals with subsequent cellular damages. This indirect effect of ionizing radiation stands for about 70% of the deleterious effects of radiation, and because of the involved pathogenic mechanisms it

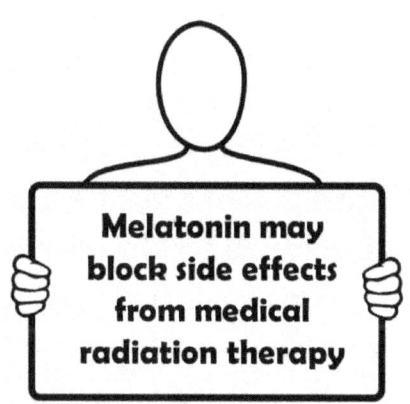

Melatonin may
block side effects
from medical
radiation therapy

would be natural to think about a strong anti-oxidant as an effective preventive treatment.

Radiation is used routinely in clinical oncology against numerous types of cancers and radiation is very effective increasing survival in these patients. However, it is well-known that external radiation may cause significant side effects including intestinal injury and injuries to other tissues like kidneys, bone marrow, liver etc. In daily clinical practice, clinicians try their best to avoid these complications by using sophisticated techniques to concentrate the radiation dose only to the cancer tissue and trying to avoid radiation to other adjacent tissues. As surgeons, however, we have unfortunately seen numerous patients with severe intestinal injury caused by radiation, especially after radiation against pelvic/gynecological cancers where especially small bowel and the rectum may be accidentally hit by the radiation treatment. Side effects may include severe proctitis, often resistant to treatment, with severe bleeding and diarrhea as well as of course pain as a very serious side effect. The radiation injury to small bowel may cause a variety of serious side effects including strictures, fistulas, diarrhea and ileus. When operating on these patients the bowel is severely damaged and because of the surgical intervention itself numerous other complications may occur and eventually cause death in these patients. The problem is therefore extremely serious and if we in any way can counteract these side effects of external radiation it would be very positive.

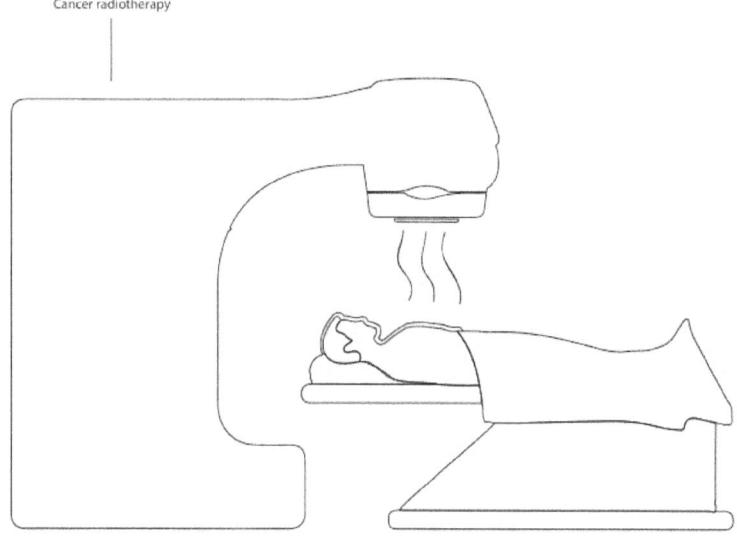

Cancer radiotherapy

In recent years, animal studies have shown extremely interesting results of using melatonin as a radio-protector. This is interesting because it can be given in a controlled manor, it has almost no side effects, is in-expensive and well tolerated. A recent study in mice found that pre-treatment with melatonin before whole body radiation treatment could very effectively counteract the effects of radiation on intestinal injury. This is fantastic medical news that warrants testing in the human clinical situation. We therefore await the results of clinical trials of the preventive effects of oral melatonin against intestinal injury caused by external radiation for cancer in the abdomen. It must be emphasized that there are absolutely no data in the literature where melatonin have shown to have negative effects in this situation and all published papers on the effects of melatonin against radiation injury have shown positive results. This includes effects on bowel injury, liver, bone marrow, kidneys, etc.

ANTI-AGING PROPERTIES OF MELATONIN - CAN MELATONIN EXTEND LIFE?

Animal experiments dating back to the 1980'ies have found an average of 20% increase in life longevity in mice with melatonin treatment. The mice were given melatonin in their nightly drinking water and the mice treated with melatonin lived on average 20% longer than the mice given normal drinking water in the evening. There are no similar data from human studies and although thousands of people or even more are taken melatonin every night we cannot expect data from this intervention until several decades from now.

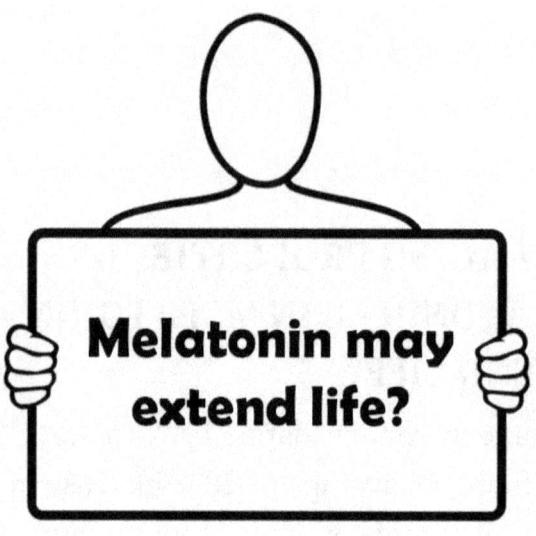

Melatonin may extend life?

The reason behind the possible increased life expectancy with external administration of melatonin may be by numerous different mechanisms. The most important possible mechanism would probably be the very intense antioxidant properties of melatonin by scavenging free oxygen radicals produced in the cells. The exact mechanism behind cell aging has not been established and this is why we cannot in detail explain the mechanism of action of melatonin in increasing life expectancy. Some of the hypotheses of normal cell aging and cell death include changes caused by free oxygen radicals in the cells and therefore melatonin may play a role in extending the cell life.

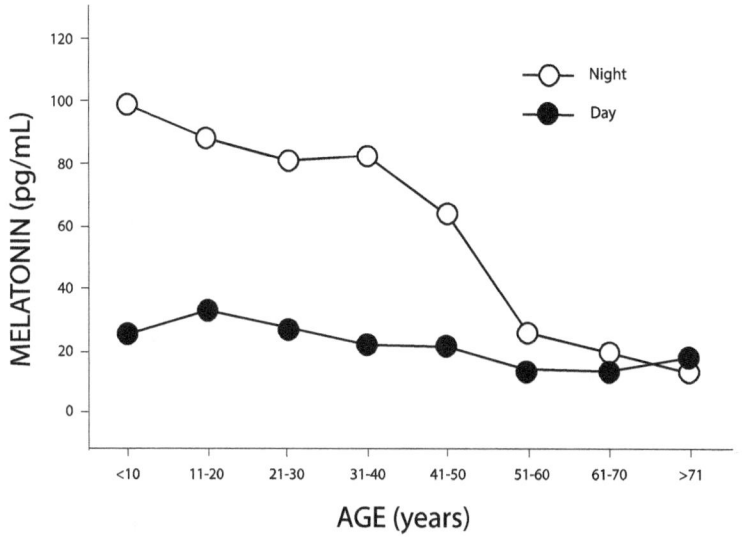

Melatonin levels decrease with age (see figure). It has therefore been hypothesized that the reduction of melatonin levels with age contributes to the aging process.

Another effective intervention in animals to increase life span is to reduce caloric intake by 40% and this has been proven to prolong life in mice, rats, dogs and monkeys by up to 30-50%. At the same time it has in fact also been shown that such a reduction in caloric intake will increase internal melatonin production that could be a possible explanation behind the observed extended life span in animals on reduced caloric intake. So it seems that we can chose between being hungry or taking melatonin tablets in the evening. You can choose for yourself what you would prefer…

Melatonin can probably be an important factor in determining the rate of aging by the ability to scavenge free oxygen radicals. These free radicals significantly affect cell-DNA and other macromolecules in the cells and melatonin administration will prevent these intracellular damages from free radicals. As discussed in another chapter of this book melatonin can effectively prevent a number of neurodegenerative diseases. Thus, it has been shown to be very effective against experimental models of Alzheimer disease as well as Parkinson's disease. In a previous very interesting case report monozygotic twins with Alzheimer's disease were treated with melatonin, but only one of the twins received melatonin. Both were followed for 3 years where one of the monozygotic twin brothers received daily melatonin. The treated brother has significantly less symptoms from Alzheimer's disease compared with his non-treated twin. Melatonin has also been shown to be effective in mild cognitive impairment as well as in more severe cases of dementia. The neurodegenerative diseases are signs of aging and melatonin seems very effective in these situations.

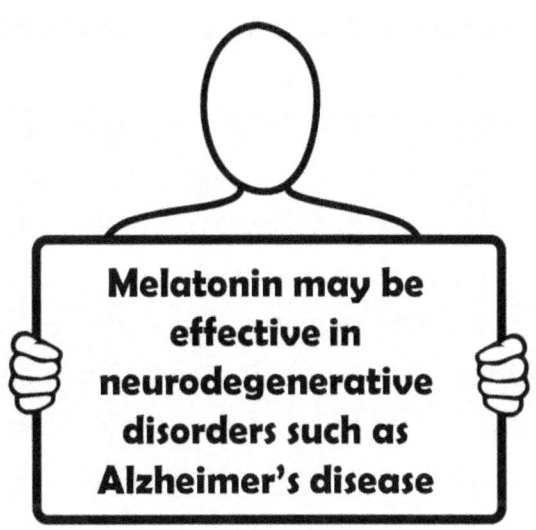

Melatonin may be effective in neurodegenerative disorders such as Alzheimer's disease

Melatonin against skin aging

Skin aging is primarily due to UV-induced cell damages in the different levels of human skin. There are different cell types that will suffer from UV damage and they include fibroblasts and keratinocytes. Very interesting experimental studies have shown that exactly these cell types are protected against UV-induced cell damage if they are pre-treated with melatonin. Thus, pre-treated cells will not die at the same rate as cells not treated with melatonin. A study found, that in UV-exposed fibroblasts only 56% of the cells survived UV exposure while cells pretreated with melatonin had a cell survival of 92.5%. The mechanism for the effect of melatonin against cell death of fibroblasts and keratinocytes is multi-factorial and includes scavenging of free oxygen radicals as well as down-regulating the expression of certain genes playing important roles in the execution of UV-induced skin photo-damage. Topical application might be meaningful since melatonin can penetrate into the skin and there build up a depot so that the action may be prolonged with topically applied melatonin in cream formulations compared with oral administration.

Theoretically, the effect of exogenous melatonin on skin aging would be effective against skin cancers and other age dependent circumstances in the skin. This will also include the development of wrinkles but this has not been shown in research studies yet.

MELATONIN – PRACTICAL DOSING

Safety

Thousands of people have participated in clinical trials with melatonin in various doses. In humans doses up to grams have been administered without side effects. With all drug testing for toxicity the so-called lethal dose (LD50) is measured. This means the dose where 50% of the test-animals die. Such studies have shown remarkable results because it has actually been impossible to establish the LD50-value for melatonin. This means, that it is impossible to kill an animal with external administration of melatonin. This is quite outstanding

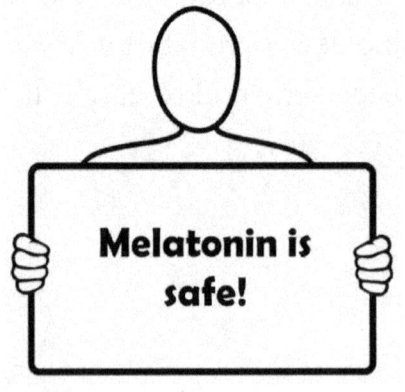

compared to all other drugs on the market where LD50 values are quite easily established.

The most common side effect seen with administration of melatonin is a slight sedative effect. However, the drug is typically taken at night time, when going to bed, so this is actually a preferred effect of melatonin and should not be considered a side-effect. Very few people take melatonin during daytime and this cannot in general be recommended because it theoretically could have an effect on e.g. driving or using machines etc. A human study where patients were given as much as 6,000 mg nightly for one month showed that some of the subjects complained of abdominal discomfort. However the side effect was transient and mild and a dose of 6,000 mg nightly can of course not be recommended for every day administration. When this is said, it should be stressed, that there are no data on effect of external melatonin in pregnant women and it should therefore probably be avoided during pregnancy and maybe also lactation where there are also no data available.

Addiction and tolerance

An amazing thing with melatonin is that there is no proof of addiction when taking this drug. Tolerance does not seem to develop and there are no withdrawal symptoms. Normally, when taking a formal sleeping agent they are typically withdrawal symptoms on the night after discontinuation of medication with very poor sleep. This is not the case with melatonin.

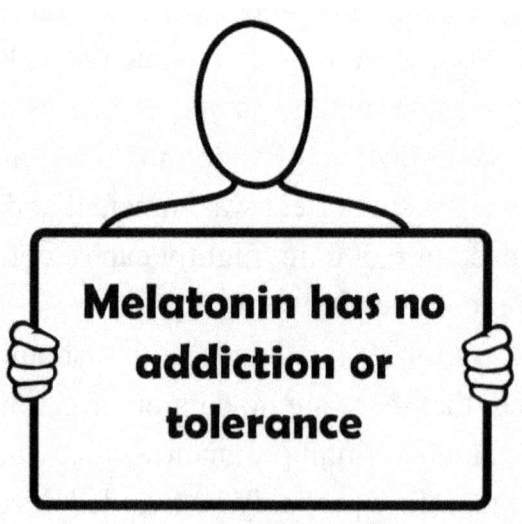

Dosing

Most people will experience a good sleep-inducing effect of only 3 mg taken at bed-time. When taking melatonin for jetlag some people will experience the need for a slightly higher dose. When taking melatonin for its antioxidant properties the dose may have to be even higher than that and dosing in the range of 20-50 mg every night would probably be in the range where antioxidant properties would be most effective.

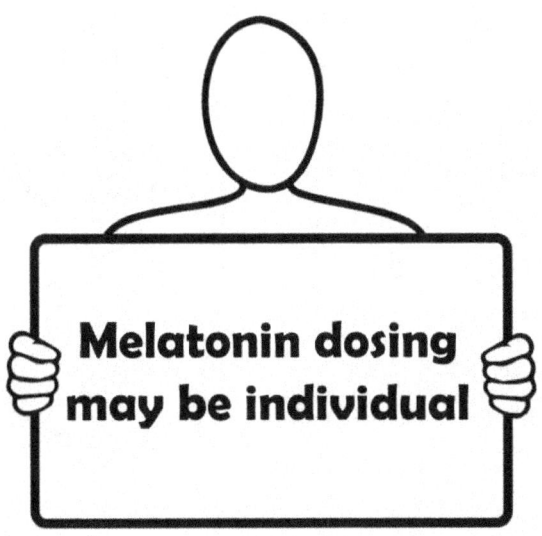

This is, however, purely hypothetical as there are no good human data to support an exact dosing regimen for its antioxidant properties, anti-aging etc. A good advice would therefore be to take a dose where you feel comfortable and where you can experience its beneficial effect on sleep and circadian rhythm.

Where do I get it?

In the US melatonin is sold in supermarkets and drug stores etc. as a vitamin-supplement. There are numerous different formulations available including "natural" melatonin, synthetic melatonin, sublingual formulations etc. It is also possible to buy slow-release 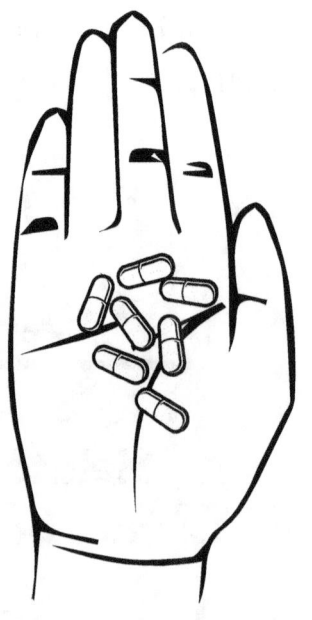 formulations of melatonin where the drug is eluted slowly during the night and not all metabolized during the first few hours of sleep. The normal half-life of melatonin is quite short so a 3 mg tablet will be metabolized quickly and there will be no more drugs left in the middle of the night. If you experience impaired sleep especially in the middle and late night hours it may be an advantage for you to take a slow release formulation of melatonin rather than the normal fast-acting drug. The sublingual formulations have their advantage in reaching higher serum-levels compared with oral intake because of the first pass effect (metabolism in the liver) with normal oral intake. However, you might as well take a higher oral dose and then still reach the same clinical effect. Melatonin is also available now even in wine gums etc. and this can be regarded as just another way to wrap the drug for normal oral intake.

SHOULD I TAKE MELATONIN?

As discussed in the previous chapters in this book there seems to be in fact only positive effects of melatonin and it is at the same time cheap and non-toxic. It therefore seems justified to consider taking melatonin every night even though you are currently healthy and without any diseases. Taking melatonin should not be done for acute relief of diseases but should more be seen as a preventive measure against long-term age-dependent deterioration such as prevention of neurodegenerative diseases, cancer, mental depression, etc. There are numerous positive clinical effects including better immune function, very effective anti-oxidant properties, effect against jet lag and insomnia, and a general anti-aging effect where it can be expected to have actually a life-extending effect, although not shown in final clinical studies yet. It is therefore hard to be critical about daily intake of exogenous melatonin. Saying that, it should of course be emphasized that we do not have data like fifty years follow up of chronic daily use in humans, but millions of doses have been administered already and there are no reported serious side effects. This is remarkable and held together with all the positive effects, both solid proven effects and potential effects based on human studies, it would be natural to consider a daily bedtime dose of melatonin.

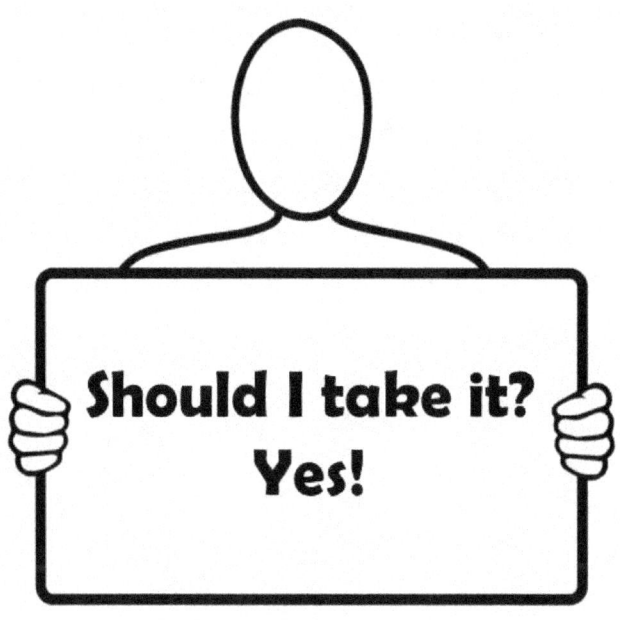

Should I take it?
Yes!

ABOUT THE AUTHORS

The authors, professor Ismail Gögenur and professor Jacob Rosenberg, are well known scientists within the effects of melatonin on various organ functions. They have studied the effects of melatonin in different clinical scenarios for the past decade and have mentored several PhD theses in this clinical field. They are based in Copenhagen, Denmark, with research collaborators all over the world.